Older People and Migration

Challenges for social work

Edited by
Susan Lawrence and Sandra Torres

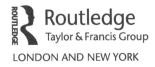

Routledge
Taylor & Francis Group

LONDON AND NEW YORK

First published 2016
by Routledge

2 Park Square, Milton Park, Abingdon, Oxon OX14 4RN
711 Third Avenue, New York, NY 10017, USA

Routledge is an imprint of the Taylor & Francis Group, an informa business

First issued in paperback 2017

British Library Cataloguing in Publication Data
A catalogue record for this book is available from the British Library

ISBN 13: 978-1-138-93550-1 (hbk)
ISBN 13: 978-1-138-09898-5 (pbk)

Typeset in Minion
by RefineCatch Limited, Bungay, Suffolk

Publisher's Note
The publisher accepts responsibility for any inconsistencies that may have
arisen during the conversion of this book from journal articles to book chapters,
namely the possible inclusion of journal terminology.

Disclaimer
Every effort has been made to contact copyright holders for their permission to
reprint material in this book. The publishers would be grateful to hear from any
copyright holder who is not here acknowledged and will undertake to rectify
any errors or omissions in future editions of this book.

Older People and Migration

With neo-liberal resource rationing, and the onus of cost shifting from the state to individuals, families, and communities, migration issues can add a further layer of complexity to the question of caring for the elderly. By presenting examples from a variety of contexts and countries, this book will stimulate readers into considering new approaches to their own local situation in an attempt to find sustainable social work responses, and in helping to build intergenerational solidarity and social capital.

Contributions to the book focus on patterns of migration: older migrants, migrating families and migrant carers. Facilitating and supporting social solidarity both locally and internationally requires social workers to understand the different contexts for social work with older people, both within their own country, and internationally. Central to this area of work is the promotion of values that respect differences and uphold the principles of human rights and social justice. This book highlights the need to consider migration as a driver for social change, offering the opportunity for new forms of social solidarity that can adapt and support people inter-generationally and sustainably in later life.

This book was originally published as a special issue of the *European Journal of Social Work*.

Susan Lawrence was President of the European Association of Schools of Social Work (EASSW) and Regional Vice President of the International Association of Schools of Social Work (IASSW) from 2011 until 2015; and until 2013 was Head of Social Work at London Metropolitan University, UK. She qualified as a Social Worker in 1976 and has been a social work academic since 1991.

Sandra Torres is Professor of Sociology and Chair in Social Gerontology at Uppsala University, Sweden. Her research—which often lies at the intersection between the sociology of ageing and the sociology of migration and ethnic relations—problematizes old age-related constructs, sheds critical light on commonly used methods in health and social care, and deconstructs some of the assumptions that guide policy and practice for the older segments of our populations.

Contents

Citation Information

The chapters in this book were originally published in the *European Journal of Social Work*, volume 15, issue 1 (February 2012). When citing this material, please use the original page numbering for each article, as follows:

Editorial

An introduction to 'the age of migration' and its consequences for the field of gerontological social work
Sandra Torres & Susan Lawrence
European Journal of Social Work, volume 15, issue 1 (February 2012) pp. 1–7

Chapter 1

The impact of migrant work in the elder care sector: recent trends and empirical evidence in Italy
Mirko Di Rosa, Maria G. Melchiorre, Maria Lucchetti & Giovanni Lamura
European Journal of Social Work, volume 15, issue 1 (February 2012) pp. 9–27

Chapter 2

Migrant workers in eldercare in Israel: social and legal aspects
Esther Iecovich & Israel Doron
European Journal of Social Work, volume 15, issue 1 (February 2012) pp. 29–44

Chapter 3

Towards a model of externalisation and denationalisation of care? The role of female migrant care workers for dependent older people in Spain
Belén Agrela Romero
European Journal of Social Work, volume 15, issue 1 (February 2012) pp. 45–61

Chapter 4

Grandmothers as main caregivers in the context of parental migration
Maria-Carmen Pantea
European Journal of Social Work, volume 15, issue 1 (February 2012) pp. 63–80

For any permission-related enquiries please visit:
http://www.tandfonline.com/page/help/permissions

Notes on Contributors

Claudio Bolzman is Professor in the Department of Social Work at the University of Applied Sciences of Western Switzerland, Geneva, Switzerland.

Mima Cattan is Professor of Public Health at the University of Northumbria, Newcastle, UK.

Mirko Di Rosa is a Postdoctoral Research Fellow at the National Institute of Health and Science on Aging, Ancona, Italy.

Israel Doron is based in the School of Social Work and Department of Gerontology at the University of Haifa, Israel.

Emilia Forssell is a Lecturer in the Institute of Social Work at Ersta Sköndal University College, Stockholm, Sweden.

Gianfranco Giuntoli holds a Research Fellowship at the Centre for Health Promotion Research at Leeds Beckett University, Leeds, UK.

Esther Iecovich is a Faculty Member in the Department of Sociology of Health and Gerontology at Ben-Gurion University of the Negev, Beer-Sheva, Israel.

Giovanni Lamura is a Senior Researcher at the National Institute of Health and Science on Aging, Ancona, Italy.

Susan Lawrence was President of the European Association of Schools of Social Work (EASSW) and Regional Vice President of the International Association of Schools of Social Work (IASSW) from 2011 until 2015; and until 2013 was Head of Social Work at London Metropolitan University, UK. She qualified as a Social Worker in 1976 and has been a social work academic since 1991.

Maria Lucchetti is based at the National Institute of Health and Science on Aging, Ancona, Italy.

Wendy Martin is Programme Leader for MSc Public Health and Health Promotion—Health Studies at Brunel University, Uxbridge, UK.

Maria G. Melchiorre is a Researcher at the National Institute of Health and Science on Aging, Ancona, Italy.

Maria-Carmen Pantea is a Professor in the Department of Social Work at Babeş-Bolyai University, Cluj-Napoca, Romania.

Belén Agrela Romero is a Professor in the Department of Physiology at the University of Jaén, Spain.

Sandra Torres is Professor of Sociology and Chair in Social Gerontology at Uppsala University, Sweden. Her research—which often lies at the intersection between the sociology of ageing and the sociology of migration and ethnic relations—problematizes old age-related constructs, sheds critical light on commonly used methods in health and social care, and deconstructs some of the assumptions that guide policy and practice for the older segments of our populations.

Christina R. Victor is Professor of Public Health in the School of Health Sciences and Social Care at Brunel University, Uxbridge, UK.

Maria Zubair is a Research Fellow in the School of Sociology and Social Policy at the University of Nottingham, UK.

An introduction to 'the age of migration' and its consequences for the field of gerontological social work

Introduction

This editorial article aims to give an introduction to the topics with which this issue is concerned by giving both an abridged presentation of 'the age of migration' and by drawing attention to some of the implications that this phenomenon has for the field of social work. As an editorial, this piece also aims to introduce the articles that comprise this special issue in an attempt to give an overview of the wide scope of topics that they touch upon. Of interest is perhaps that when we first agreed to act as guest editors to this special issue we were primarily thinking that most of the articles we were going to publish were going to be about older people per se. The wide range of issues that the articles in this special issue cover suggest, however, that 'the age of migration' is challenging gerontological social work in more ways than we might initially imagine.

This special issue is, in other words, far more diverse than we first expected it to be. As such, it is a true testament to the many challenges that 'the age of migration' poses to social work research, practice and education as well as to social policy. It is for this reason that we decided to use the social scientific debate on the globalization of international migration in our editorial—albeit in an abridged form—as a frame of reference when describing the articles that follow. This special issue aims ultimately to raise awareness of the increasing need to develop social work practices that are not only old age-sensitive but also international migration-aware.

Globalization as a backdrop

In one of the latest additions to the textbook literature on introductions to social work, Wilson *et al.* (2008) summarize the challenges that our field faces in the twenty-first century by writing that:

> The trend towards an ageing population and the consequent declining tax base will mean that social work and social care with older people/.../ will be an expanding and increasingly controversial area of practice and policy. Changing patterns of international migration associated with global economic inequalities, post-conflict dispersion of ethnic groups, and the shifting balance of socio-economic power among nations and continents, are likely to result in social work with asylum seekers, immigrants, people that have been trafficked, and people who are part of the 'grey economy' becoming an increasing focus of need and intervention. (p. 654)

This assessment is in line with what social scientists around the world have argued when they have tried to draw attention to the fact that the globalization of international migration is posing numerous challenges to our societies. This is the case because 'the global order based on sovereign national states is giving way to something new' (Castles & Miller, 2003, p. 1). That something new—which we call globalization—is bringing about the growth of interactions between a range of social, economic, and cultural networks across the world. In this respect it seems important to acknowledge that although the debate on globalization within social work has not been as lively as it has been in other social scientific areas there are in fact some social work theorists that have discussed the implications of globalization for social work practice (e.g. Lister, 1998; Khan & Dominelli, 2000; Penna et al., 2000; Pugh & Gould, 2000; Ahmadi, 2003; Webb, 2003; Lyons, 2006; Midgley, 2006; Lawrence et al., 2009).

Among the transformations that have been identified as constitutive features of globalization processes are the geographical expansion and increased density of international trade; the development of a worldwide capitalist economy and of multinational corporations; the emergence of what Beck (2000, p. 11) calls 'polycentric world politics'; the dispersion of mass media across the world; and the variety of innovations that have taken place in information and telecommunications technology. In addition to this we have the transnational actors, communities, social spaces, and structures that these transformations imply. These have all brought about a variety of worldwide exchanges that have made the transcendence of traditional national boundaries possible. It is because of all of this that Archer (1990) has argued that globalization is affecting every major aspect of social reality to such an extent that some have suggested that we are experiencing the end of the world as we know it. To this end, Smart (1993) has asserted that our understanding of what is meant by 'society' and where the boundaries should be drawn when we talk about what is deemed 'social' is being challenged by the fact that the new geopolitical order does not really resemble the modern nation-state. Irrespective of the various sources of questioning that one can employ in order to raise doubt about the origins and scope of globalization, there is a growing awareness within social work that 'globalization has some descriptive merit' (Pugh & Gould, 2000, p. 136).

Although we agree to a certain extent with Pugh and Gould's (2000) assessment that there is a risk that the 'omnipresence of the term (globalization) contributes much to the "taken-for-granted" acceptance of the idea' (Pugh & Gould, 2000, p. 124) and with their assertion that it is problematic to regard globalization as a phenomenon that will inevitably dismantle welfare service, we cautiously propose that failure to acknowledge the challenges posed by globalization could lead to the disempowerment of our field. Hence, that we 'accept the descriptive use of globalization as a means of referring to the social and economic changes' (Pugh & Gould, p. 2000) that are taking place and find the debate on the globalization of international migration to be particularly useful as a frame of reference for this introduction. It is, after all, the very 'age of migration' that most likely lead this journal's editor-in-chief to commission this special issue. The globalization of international migration is one of the phenomena (population ageing being another) that poses the kind of 'challenges from the margins' that Khan and Dominelli (2000) argue to be at the very core of what makes globalization a force with which social work must reckon.

With regard to the time of the life-course with which this special issue is concerned (i.e. old age) it has elsewhere been argued that globalization is challenging not only the way in which we study old age but also the manner in which we think about older migrants (e.g. Torres, 2006a). With regard to the former, Phillipson (2007) has argued that 'globalization has emerged as a transformative force, reshaping the boundaries within which old age is experienced' (p. 291). In a similar vein, Warnes *et al.* (2004) have argued that the globalization of international migration is as important to the study of old age and ageing as population ageing is.[1] The age of migration can affect the study of ageing and old age in numerous ways, and population ageing has actualized the need to develop a gerontological social work for the twenty-first century. This is why there is a need for a special issue such as this one; an issue that draws attention to some of the challenges to social work practice with older people that the globalization of international migration poses.

What does the 'the age of migration' mean and why should social workers care?

The age of migration was the title of a book about the consequences for society of global migration flows (Castles & Miller, 2003). This book is considered to be a seminal work by international migration and ethnic relations researchers since it gave an overview of the scope and patterns of international migration flows across the world and considered the various implications that these flows have for the ethnic composition of different societies. Although some demographers have questioned whether or not we can speak of the twentieth century as the age of migration, their own calculations confirm that the migrant stock has increased tremendously over the past four decades (Zlotnik, 1999). Therefore, it seems important to acknowledge that although we may question whether the age of migration is really as wide a global trend as Castles and Miller (2003) have suggested, it is clear that the globalization of international migration has, as a social phenomenon, affected the West in general and Europe in particular in an indisputable way (cf. Castles, 2000a; Okólski, 2000). In this respect, Zlotnik (1999) shows that both North America and Western Europe have experienced higher rates of migrant stock during the past four decades. They argue, therefore, that 'the international migration experience of countries in the West not only exerts considerable weight in global trends but is also instrumental in influencing general perceptions of the phenomenon' (Zlotnik, 1999, p. 24).

It is this type of upswing in migration flows that has led some scholars to refer to the EU as a de facto region of immigration (e.g. Muus, 2001). One of the issues that Castles and Miller (2003) brought to the fore is how certain general tendencies that have arisen over the past two decades specifically[2] have led to a state of affairs in which few societies are exempted from this phenomenon. They argue that more and more countries are nowadays affected by international migration, which is why it has become difficult to draw a line between immigration and emigration countries. This has led to an increase in the awareness by policy-makers at the domestic, regional, and national level that international migration is a phenomenon they must reckon with. As Ahmadi (2003) has stated with respect to international social work in particular: 'international migration makes poverty, political and religious oppression, and the lack of civil rights in one society the concern of other societies' (Ahmadi, 2003, p. 15).

The two other tendencies that Castles and Miller (Ahmadi, 2003) describe as characteristic of 'the age of migration' are the feminization and differentiation of migration. The former relates to the fact that women are now playing a central role in almost all of the migration flows that we are observing across the world, which is affecting how we think of migration and migrants. The first three articles in this special issue written by Di Rosa *et al.*, Iecovich and Doron, and Romero address this very theme. The differentiation of migration—which is also related to the issue of feminization—concerns the increasingly common phenomena of migrant care workers, typically, though not exclusively female. These three articles discuss the impact on the elders cared for and their families, on the care sector and on the migrant workers themselves in Italy, Israel, and Spain.

With respect to the differentiation of migrant flows to Europe, King (2002) has stated that migration to this region are challenging us to think of migration in new terms since the often taken-for-granted assumption that all migrants are poor and uneducated is no longer (if it ever was) applicable. It is for all of these reasons that 'the age of migration' is deemed to have unprecedented implications for all aspects of migration studies: from the way in which we used to think about distinctions between 'sending' and 'receiving' countries, as well as the stereotypical assumptions about immigrants and refugees that are often made (Richmond, 2002), to the way in which we study migration movements and their implications for national and international policies (Castles & Davidson, 2000). Even the manner in which we approach the study of migrants and policies relevant to their needs is being challenged by 'the age of migration' (Kivisto, 2001). This is why there is a need to raise social work's awareness of the challenges that the globalization of international migration poses. It is in this context that the article in this special issue by Pantea discusses the contribution made by grandmothers in Romania as full-time carers of children whose parents have migrated in search of employment. Pantea points to the stigma sometimes faced by those grandmothers and a social policy and social work system struggling with the challenge of how best to support the children left behind and their carers.

In his book on the impact of globalization on the study of ethnicity, Castles (2000b) answers the very question that is at the core of this special issue; namely why should social work care about the globalization of international migration? The answer is that migration 'is both a result of global change and a powerful source for further change in migrant-sending and receiving-societies' (Castles, 2000b, p. 124). As such, this phenomenon affects all spheres of social life and is bound to challenge social work practice. Hence that we suggest—as the articles in this special issue will show—that we are in dire need to develop social work practice that is not only old age-sensitive but international migration-aware. With respect to both of these concerns Warnes *et al.* (2004) have argued that:

> the number of older people who have been international migrants and have cultural differences from the host population have grown and will undoubtedly increase during the coming decades; and second (that) the case for a more systematic and proactive response to the problems and structured disadvantages of older migrants will become more compelling. (309–310)

The contributions by Victor *et al.*, Bolzman, Forssell, and Torres, and Giuntoli and Cattan that we have included in this special issue attest to the points that the authors quoted above make. These articles all show that older migrants are, as a social work category, a very heterogeneous group.[3] This heterogeneity—as well as the increased differentiation of migrants in all age groups—has led to an increased awareness in social policy and social work that our conceptualizations of citizenship need to be revised since they depart from ideals of equality and universality that are not compatible with the diversity and difference that characterizes our times (cf. Lister, 1998). With respect to the increasing diversity with which the age of migration is associated, Khan and Dominelli (2000) have questioned whether changes toward 'a highly procedualized and bureaucratic process of assessment' in social work are in fact compatible with the need to accommodate increasing diversity. In this respect it seems interesting to note that one of the issues often brought up when the challenges posed by globalization are being discussed is the fact that specific social work practices—such as international social work and anti-oppressive practice (AOP) and anti-discriminatory practice (ADP)—have also been developed to counteract the neo-liberalist movement that globalization is associated with. With respect to the former—that is, international social work—it is interesting to note that the need to develop social work practice that transcends national borders is often discussed when ways to meet the challenges posed by globalization are brought to fore (e.g. Ahmadi, 2003; Lyons, 2006; Midgley, 2006; Lawrence *et al.*, 2009). This is poignantly demonstrated in the contributions to this special issue made by Pantea, Lemura *et al.*, and Romero who are all—in different ways—focusing on some of the transnationalist aspects of the age of migration. As such, their work suggests—albeit in implicit ways—that international collaborations in social work practice may be needed now that the interdependence of countries is more easily tangible.[4] With respect to social work practices believed to counteract globalizing forces it seems important to draw attention to the egalitarian humanism that characterizes ADP since this one practice is believed to have the potential to become an antidote to some of the problems with which globalization is associated (cf. Penna *et al.*, 2000). The limited scope of this editorial does not allow us to discuss these issues at length. We do not aim either to suggest how the challenges hereby alluded to are best addressed. Suffice it to say that there is evidence that 'it is precisely under conditions of globalization that significant forms of solidarity have/. . ./ emerged' (Pugh & Gould, 2000, p. 137).

Notes

[1]   For insight into the debate on the impact of international migration on the advancement of the population ageing process see, for example, Bijak *et al.* (2007) and Tsimbos (2006).

[2]   Such as the fact that international migration flows have accelerated in all major regions of the world, leading not only to the globalization of this phenomenon but also to its politicization.

[3]   The issue of heterogeneity has received little attention. It is as if there is a persistent need to think of older migrants in homogenizing ways (cf. Torres, 2006b).

[4]   Hereby we acknowledge that there are some who question whether efforts to create international and/or transnational social work practices are the most suitable to address the challenges that globalization poses (e.g. Webb, 2003).

References

Ahmadi, N. (2003) 'Globalization of consciousness and new challenges for international migration', *International Journal of Social Welfare*, vol. 12, pp. 14–23.

Archer, M. (1990) 'Foreword', in *Globalization, Knowledge and Society*, eds M. Albrow & E. King, Sage, London, Thousand Oaks, New Delhi, pp. 1–3.

Beck, U. (2000) *What is Globalization?*, Polity Press, Cambridge.

Bijak, J., Kupiszewska, D., Kupiszewski, M., Saczuk, K & Kicinger, A. (2007) 'Population and labor force projections for 27 European countries, 2002–2052: impact of international migration on population ageing', *European Journal of Population*, vol. 23, no. 1, pp. 1–31.

Castles, S. (2000a) 'International migration at the beginning of the twenty-first century: global trends and issues', *International Social Science Journal*, vol. 52, no. 165, pp. 269–281.

Castles, S. (2000b) *Ethnicity and Globalization: From Migrant Worker to Transnational Citizen*, Thousand Oaks, and New Delhi, Sage, London.

Castles, S. & Davidson, A. (2000) *Citizenship and Migration: Globalization and the Politics of Belonging*, Macmillan Press Ltd, London.

Castles, S. & Miller, M. J. (2003) *The Age of Migration*, 3rd edn, Palgrave Macmillan, Basingstoke.

Khan, P. & Dominelli, L. (2000) 'The impact of globalization on social work in the UK', *European Journal of Social Work*, vol. 3, no. 2, pp. 95–108.

King, R. (2002) 'Towards a new map of European migration', *International Journal of Population Geography*, vol. 8, no. 2, pp. 89–106.

Kivisto, P. (2001) 'Theorizing transnational immigration: a critical review of current efforts', *Ethnic and Racial Studies*, vol. 24, no. 4, pp. 549–577.

Lawrence, S., Lyons, K., Simpson, G. & Huegler, N. (eds) (2009) *Introducing International Social Work*, Learning Matters, Exeter.

Lister, R. (1998) 'Citizenship on the margins: citizenship, social work and social action', *European Journal of Social Work*, vol. 1, no. 1, pp. 5–18.

Lyons, K. (2006) 'Globalization and social work: international and local implications', *British Journal of Social Work*, vol. 36, pp. 365–380.

Midgley, J. (2006) 'International social work, globalization and the challenge of a unipolar world', *Journal of Sociology and Social Welfare*, vol. 33, no. 4, pp. 11–17.

Muus, P. (2001) 'International migration and the European Union: trends and consequences', *European Journal on Criminal Policy and Research*, vol. 9, no. 1, pp. 31–49.

Okólski, H. (2000) 'Recent trends and major issues in international migration: Central and East European perspectives', *International Social Science Journal*, vol. 52, no. 165, pp. 329–342.

Penna, S., Paylor, I. & Washington, J. (2000) 'Globalization, social exclusion and the possibilities for global social work and welfare', *European Journal of Social Work*, vol. 3, no. 2, pp. 109–122.

Phillipson, C. (2007) "New ageing and new policy responses: reconstructing gerontology in a global age", in *New Dynamics in Old Age: Individual, Environmental and Societal Perspectives*, eds H.-W. Wahl, C. Tesh-Römer & A. Hoff, Baywood Publishing, Amityville, NY, pp. 291–305.

Pugh, R. & Gould, N. (2000) 'Globalization, social work and social welfare', *European Journal of Social Work*, vol. 3, no. 2, pp. 123–138.

Richmond, A. H. (2002) 'Globalization: implications for immigrants and refugees', *Ethnic and Racial Studies*, vol. 25, no. 5, pp. 707–727.

Smart, B. (1993) *Postmodernity*, Routledge, London and New York.

Torres, S. (2006a) 'Culture, migration, inequality and 'periphery' in a globalized world: challenges for ethno- and anthropogerontology', in *Ageing, Globalization and Inequality: The New Critical Gerontology*, eds J. Baars, D. Dannefer, C. Phillipson & A. Walker, Baywood Publishing, Amityville, NY.

Torres, S. (2006b) 'Elderly immigrants in Sweden: "Otherness" under construction', *Journal of Ethnic and Migration Studies*, vol. 32, no. 8, pp. 1341–1358.

Tsimbos, C. (2006) 'The impact of migration on growth and ageing of the population in a new receiving country: the case of Greece', *International Migration*, vol. 44, no. 4, pp. 231–254.

Warnes, A. M., Friedrich, K., Kellaher, L. & Torres, S. (2004) 'The diversity and welfare of older migrants in Europe', *Ageing and Society*, vol. 24, no. 3, pp. 647–663.

Webb, S. A. (2003) 'Local orders and global chaos in social work', *European Journal of Social Work*, vol. 6, no. 2, pp. 191–204.

Wilson, K., Ruch, G., Lymbery, M. & Cooper, A. (2008) *Social Work: An Introduction to Contemporary Practice*, Pearson Education Limited, Essex, England.

Zlotnik, H. (1999) 'Trends in international migration since 1965: what existing data reveal', *International Migration*, vol. 37, no. 1, pp. 21–61.

SANDRA TORRES
Uppsala University, Uppsala, Sweden
Oslo University College, Oslo, Norway
King's College London, London, UK
Swedish Gerontological Society, Uppsala, Sweden

SUSAN LAWRENCE
London Metropolitan University, London, UK
European Association of Schools of Social Work, Netherlands

The impact of migrant work in the elder care sector: recent trends and empirical evidence in Italy

L'impatto delle assistenti familiari straniere nel settore della cura agli anziani: tendenze recenti ed evidenze empiriche in Italia

Mirko Di Rosa, Maria G. Melchiorre, Maria Lucchetti & Giovanni Lamura

Italy is characterized by a very high and increasing demand for elder care but, paradoxically, also by a surprisingly low level of public service provision in this sector. Due to current demographic, economic and socio-cultural trends, the potential availability of informal family care has been decreasing while, on the other hand, still strong familistic attitudes have so far limited the emergence of formal—both home and residential—care services. The 'cash-for-care' orientation of the Italian welfare system, with direct payments prevailing over in-kind services, has thus gradually developed into a care regime where monetary transfers to dependent (older) people are often used to privately employ migrant care workers. This phenomenon is analyzed in the context of two different studies (EUROFAMCARE and DIPO), in order to understand how migrant care work has been affecting both family care and professional care work in Italy. The main findings suggest that the widespread employment of migrant care workers—propelled by public care allowances—has certainly relieved many families from most burdensome care tasks, but at the same time partly 'crowded out' formal care services. Care quality issues remain. however, largely under-investigated, as do care drain effects in sending countries.

L'Italia è caratterizzata da una domanda di assistenza agli anziani molto elevata ed in ulteriore crescita, ma, paradossalmente, anche da un livello sorprendentemente basso di fornitura di servizi pubblici in questo settore. A causa dell'attuale situazione demografica, economica e socio-culturale, la potenziale disponibilità di assistenza familiare informale appare in calo mentre, d'altro canto, l'ancor forte attitudine 'familistica' ha finora limitato l'emergere di servizi di assistenza formali, sia domiciliari che residenziali. L'orientamento 'cash-for-care' del sistema di welfare italiano, che eroga pagamenti diretti piuttosto che servizi, ha così progressivamente trasformato il sistema di assistenza nel senso di un frequente impiego dei trasferimenti monetari agli anziani non autosufficienti per l'assunzione privata di assistenti familiari straniere. Questo fenomeno è stato analizzato sulla base di due diversi studi (EUROFAMCARE e DIPO), al fine di comprendere come il lavoro di cura prestato da queste figure in Italia influisca sia sull'assistenza familiare che su quella erogata dai servizi socio-sanitari. I principali risultati ottenuti suggeriscono che il largo impiego delle collaboratrici familiari straniere—incentivato da assegni di assistenza pubblici—ha certamente sollevato molte famiglie dai compiti di supporto più onerosi, ma, allo stesso tempo, anche finito con il sostituire parzialmente i servizi formali di cura. Restano tuttavia in gran parte da approfondire i problemi legati alla qualità dell'assistenza, così come gli effetti di 'care drain' sollevati da questo fenomeno nei paesi di origine.

Introduction

Aims and structure of this article

This article analyses the phenomenon of migrant care work in the Italian elder care sector, by providing first an overview of most recent trends affecting the demand for this specific form of care work in Europe and especially in Italy, illustrated by available literature. After a short description of the methodology used to collect and analyse the data presented in this contribution—i.e. the datasets produced by the EUROFAMCARE and DIPO studies (section 2)—selected findings from these two research projects will be presented with regard to the role played by migrant workers in providing care to older people living in the community (section 3). Results will focus on the kind of activities performed by migrant care workers (MCWs)[1] and their impact on both informal and formal support resources. Main determinants of families' decision to seek the help of MCWs will be also highlighted. These findings will be discussed in section 4, together with some concluding remarks on the main challenges raised by this phenomenon, in an attempt to set an—albeit provisional—agenda for future research, policy and practice in this still largely neglected area of interest.

Migrant care work for older people: a global phenomenon

The migration of long-term (or elder) care[2] workers is an increasing, worldwide phenomenon, which reflects the in-depth changes associated with the globalization of the international economy and the growing interdependence existing between countries (Redfoot & Houser, 2005; Anderson, 2007; Brown & Braun, 2008). Its peculiarity lies in the fact that long-term elder care involves what have been called 'anchored' jobs, i.e. tasks that must be performed on a face-to-face basis and imply a direct contact with the client or patient (Friedman, 2005), and cannot be easily outsourced or relocated elsewhere from the point of delivery. The pressure to employ MCWs is thus rapidly increasing in countries where domestic labour markets cannot fill these jobs, in order to reduce care staff shortages (Holzer, 2003; European Commission, 2005). In these nations this phenomenon is likely to have an in-depth impact on traditional patterns of elder care delivery, traditionally provided by families as well as by health and social care workers both in home and residential care settings.

Migrant care work in Europe

The employment of MCWs is currently taking place on a large scale in Europe, especially—but not only—in Southern European countries (Lethbridge, 2007; European Communities, 2008; Lamura *et al.*, 2008). Care migration patterns in this geographic area have been partly fueled by public cash for care schemes providing benefits to dependent persons. These have attracted large numbers of unskilled, mainly live-in domestic workers, primarily women, who are often employed by families in a grey economy characterized by illegal immigration and/or work status. However, one main difference which can be currently observed between this more recent phenomenon taking place in Southern Europe—but increasingly also in Central European countries like Austria (Schneider & Trukeschitz, 2008) and Germany (DIP, 2009), as well as in a 'familistic' nation like Ireland (Timonen *et al.*, 2006)—and the care migration patterns characterizing Northern Europe is that foreign-born workers in the latter area are more frequently employed by formal care service providers, rather than—on a private basis—by families (Figure 1). This is clearly reflected by the fact that the percentage of migrants employed in care services appears to be the highest in countries like the UK, Sweden and Norway, where the majority of them are employed in community services, and are also likely to be represented not by newcomers, but rather by long-settled migrants, who end up working in this sector later on in their migration career.

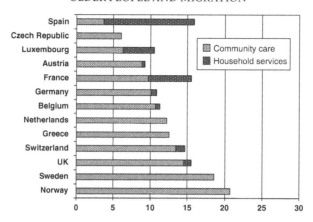

Figure 1 Foreign-born workers in community and household services (%).

In Mediterranean countries, on the contrary, the private employment of MCWs by families has today become the 'normal' solution to face the elder care challenge. Figures—despite the limitations due to the high degree of undeclared work, which makes official statistics often unreliable in this field—are striking: in Greece one-fourth of all migrants (but 80% of migrant women!) are estimated to be employed in personal care/household services (Kavounidi, 2004); in Spain the number of permits for domestic work to foreigners rose from 33,000 in 1999 to almost 230,000 in 2006 (INE, 2008); in Turkey the employment of Moldovan and Bulgarian domestic workers has become the rule in private households (Kaska, 2006 cited in Suter, 2008). In some cases the phenomenon has been legitimized by long term care insurance (LTCI) schemes, such as in Israel—where about one out of three frail elderly persons is currently cared for by a migrant live—in homecare worker employed through such a scheme (Iecovich, 2009)—and even in Austria where, in the light of a generous LTCI—containing specific provisions to recognize and facilitate the employment of migrant workers—today over 20% of all care workers have a migration background (Schneider & Trukeschitz, 2008).

The role of migrant care work in the Italian welfare system

With almost 20% of its population aged 65 years or older (US Census Bureau, 2008), Italy represents today one of the oldest countries in the world, and estimates indicate that this age group will grow up to almost one-third of the whole population by 2040 (Eurostat, 2007a). At the same time, three parallel phenomena are potentially affecting in negative terms the availability of informal carers in Italy. The first concerns the decreasing 'potential support ratio' (between the number of adults of working age, 15–64, and the number of older people aged over 65), which with about three adults per older person is already very low in Italy if compared to other countries (UN, 2006). A further trend is represented by the increased female participation rate in the labour market (i.e. the ratio between the female labour force of all ages and the female population aged 15–64), which between 1994 and 2004 increased from 42.4% to 51% (OECD, 2005), and recently even beyond (ISTAT, 2008). Parallel to this, a perceptible delay in the time of retirement is taking place following a series of pension reforms, as shown by the fact that in 2006 the employment rate in the 55–64-year-old age group—the one in which many informal carers of older people are also traditionally concentrated—reached 32.5% (Eurostat, 2007b), five points higher than in 2000, although still remaining one of the lowest in Europe (Aliaga & Romans, 2006).

These changes are challenging the traditional pattern followed by the Italian welfare state, mainly based on a substantial contribution of unpaid family support to grant long-term care to dependent elderly, so that an increasing number of Italian households have been trying to face this task by privately employing migrants, often on a live-in basis, as home care workers. Several pull factors have operated to attract this workforce to Italy—besides the above-mentioned decrease in the availability of informal carers—such as a traditional preference for care payments (rather than direct care services), the cultural vision that elderly care is to a large extent a 'family matter', and the related aversion to residential care. Compared to most Europeans, Italians still maintain indeed a relatively 'familistic' approach toward elder care, as reflected by the above-average percentages (25%, compared to an EU-25 level of 18%) of Italians holding that 'children should pay for the care of their own parents', or considering it a 'good thing if in the future working adults would have to look after their elderly parents more than they do nowadays' (75% vs. an EU-25 average of 42%) (Alber & Köhler, 2004). Under such circumstances, it is not surprising that, within Europe, Italy reports one of the highest percentages of women aged 55–64 who are 'inactive' in the labour market because of family responsibilities (30% of all women, compared to an EU-15 average of 10%) (Van Bastelaer & Blöndal, 2003).

At the same time, the role of formal care services remains underdeveloped and unequally distributed throughout the country. Home care services reach only 4.9% of the over-65-year-old population, and are mostly concentrated in northern regions (Gori & Casanova, 2009). A similar, unequal distribution penalizing southern areas is true for residential care facilities, which host no more than 3% of the total number of older Italians, a percentage which has remained stable in the last decade (Pesaresi & Brizioli, 2009). Parallel to this, a cost-driven rationalization of health care processes has determined a remarkable shortening in the average length of hospital stays (Ministero della Salute, 2000–2007), thus producing, as a consequence, an increase in the number of inappropriate, untimely 'allocations' of especially older patients in residential care facilities (Tinti, 2004). On the whole, the very high rate of physicians (4.2 per 1000 inhabitants), compared to a relatively low presence of nurses (5.4 per 1000 inhabitants) (WHO, 2006), reflects a longstanding shortage of nursing staff, and the lack of measures to shift resources from the acute care to the long-term care sector.

The marginal role of Italian formal elder care services finds an even clearer explanation in light of a further, basic characteristic of the Italian welfare state: its 'cash-for-care' orientation, i.e. the traditional predominance of care payments, rather than of in-kind services. Dependent persons in Italy are indeed entitled to receive the following, different care payments: (a) a means-tested *disability pension* by the State, which reaches 255 Euros per month; (b) a *care allowance*, also by the State, which is not means-tested and amounts to 472 Euros per month (756 Euros in case of blindness); and (c) *cash benefits*, introduced more recently by some local authorities, which are usually means-tested and do not exceed 300–500 Euros per month. Summing up the different types of care payments, a total sum of 700–900 Euros per month therefore becomes available to recipients who can count on at least two of the above care payments (i.e. a sum that is not far away from the average income of an over-65-year-old Italian living alone). Due to a lack of controls,[3] however, especially the State care allowance has reached a very wide audience—currently amounting to circa 9.5% of all over-65-year-old Italians, up from 5.5% in 2001 (Lamura & Principi, 2009)—thus becoming a hidden form of income integration, partly as a result of local 'clientelism' phenomena (Lamura *et al.*, 2001).

In light of the developments outlined above, it is therefore not surprising that an increasing number of Italian families have turned to MCWs to provide care to their frail older members. Official statistics reflect quite clearly this phenomenon: while in 1991 only 16% of the 181,000 domestic care workers recorded at that time had a foreign nationality (INPS, 1992), current estimates speak of 72% foreign-born persons among the now almost 1,485,000 persons employed in a sector which has experienced an enormous growth (37% in only the past 7 years) (CENSIS, 2009). A large number of these MCWs, mainly women, live with the persons they care for, and come mainly from Eastern Europe—in particular from Ukraine and Romania, but also from Poland, Moldova and Albania—although a considerable number of them are from South America and Asiatic countries like the Philippines and Sri Lanka (INPS-Caritas/Migrantes, 2004).

If we consider only households directly involved in providing informal care to a dependent older person, 13% of them report privately employing a paid care worker (Lamura *et al.*, 2008). Households who are most likely to resort to this solution are those that are involved in heavy care tasks, such as providing assistance to a demented family member (more than one out of four Italian families facing this challenge employ a MCW) or a severely disabled one (more than one-third of these). This is a clear indicator of the fact that the private employment of care migrants has become a systematic solution in Italy to tackle long-term care needs, when these cannot be properly met by traditional home and residential care services.

In the light of the above observation, it is therefore crucial to understand how the help provided by privately hired MCWs has changed the role played by the family and formal care services. In the following analysis this will be investigated by identifying which tasks are mainly delegated to MCWs and which are retained by traditional care providers, distinguishing between live-in and non-live-in situations. Furthermore, a more in-depth analysis of the main factors affecting families' decision to employ a

MCW, on the one hand, as well as of the MCW's long-term perspectives, on the other hand, will provide insight on the sustainability of this solution for the future.

Methodology

The analysis presented here has been based on two studies carried out in Italy in 2004–2005. The first one concerns the Italian section of EUROFAMCARE, a broad survey carried out in six European countries on family caregiving, in which some questions on migrant care work were added to the common research protocol and administered to Italian respondents only. The second study (DIPO) refers to a regional investigation conducted in Central Italy and specifically aimed at collecting in-depth information on MCWs. Some of the questions posed were the same in both studies, whose design is briefly described in the following.

The EUROFAMCARE study[4]

The Italian survey for the EUROFAMCARE study reached 990 family caregivers of older people who—in accordance to the European investigation's aims—were interviewed in order to evaluate the availability and use of services providing support and respite to carers. Following a protocol for sample selection and recruitment agreed with the other European partners, respondents were administered a quantitative Common Assessment Tool (CAT) through face-to-face interviews. The questionnaire used for the Italian survey included, as an appendix to the CAT, a few questions focused on the topic of migrant care work, investigating whether this source of support was used by families to provide elder care, for which tasks and under which circumstances (i.e. whether the MCW was living in or not with the older person to be cared for). A total of 129 families—i.e. 13% of the 990 representing the overall Italian sample—reported to be employing a MCW at the moment of the data collection.

The DIPO study[5]

This survey was conducted in the region of Marche (Central Italy) on a sample of 220 foreign women privately employed by families in order to provide care to their older members. Subjects were recruited in two different areas—one city in the coastal area and one in a mixed (urban-rural) area in the mountainous hinterland—through snowballing techniques via local migrants associations, in an attempt to 'capture' both migrants regularly employed and those working as undeclared care staff (i.e. without legal permit of stay nor/or a working permit).

A structured questionnaire was administered face-to-face, focussing on living and working conditions of migrant women engaged in care activities to support dependent older people, with the aim of understanding whether and to what extent migrant care work is supplementing/replacing care provided by the family as well as by other formal (public, private or voluntary) care service providers.

Data analysis

Data from both studies were first analysed to obtain basic, descriptive information on the main tasks performed by MCWs, according to their (non) live-in status. A comparison between the tasks performed by the MCWs, by the family and by formal care providers was then carried out, in order to highlight the impact exerted by MCWs on the role played by the other (both formal and informal) care providers.

The EUROFAMCARE study included information on both family carers and MCWs, thus allowing us to compare families employing MCWs with families not relying on them. This latter group was not included in the DIPO study, which therefore provides only information on the different role played by MCWs according to their (non) live-in status. On the other hand, the DIPO dataset allows us to capture the MCWs' opinion on the long-term sustainability of this solution.

Finally, a logistic regression was performed to identify the main features characterising the families who decide to employ a MCW. This model was chosen since it can be applied to dichotomous dependent variables (such as in this case), and to identify not only which variables significantly affect the dependent one, but also (through the odds ratio) in which proportion. The logistic regression included the following variables: (1) characteristics of the caregiver (employment status; gender; marital status; kin relationship to the cared-for older person; living distance from older person; type of work; emotional relationship to the older person); (2) characteristics of the older person (hours of care per week; length of caregiving period; degree of dependence); (3) available support (presence of a network enabling the carer to have a break; types of most relevant supports; features of the most important support). The validity and overall reliability of the model was assessed by means of diagnostic tests such as the F-test of joint '0' coefficients R-square, the Hosmer–Lemeshow and the estimation of the area beneath the ROC curve.

Findings: the impact of migrant care work on family and professional care of older people

Care tasks carried out by migrant care workers

Italian families providing care to dependent older people employ MCWs mainly to receive support in terms of housework, preparation and administration of meals, company and personal care (Table 1). On the other hand, the tasks which MCWs are least frequently in charge of are management of finances, organization of care and transportation, which remain mainly a 'family affair'. An intermediate position characterizes activities such as the administration of medicines, lifting the older person and/or helping her/him to move at home and the accomplishment of external tasks (such as, for instance, shopping), all tasks whose frequency increases remarkably only in cases where the MCW lives in with the older person. Living in represents indeed a condition which is associated with a more frequent involvement of MCWs

Table 1 Care tasks performed by migrant workers privately employed by families of dependent older people, by (non)living in status (%)

	Eurofamcare		Dipo	
	Live-in	Non-live-in	Live-in	Non-live-in
Care task	n = 84	n = 29	n = 126	n = 94
Housework	98.8	89.7	86.5	72.3
Meals preparation/administration	94.1	65.5	85.7	60.6
Company	84.5	72.4	84.9	74.5
Personal care and hygiene	82.1	72.4	90.5	80.9
Medicines administration	85.7	58.6	59.5	44.7
Lifting/moving at home	81.0	65.5	63.5	41.5
Shopping	58.3	41.4	61.9	36.2
Transportation	17.1	27.6	50.8	35.1
Organization of care	12.2	20.7	_a	_a
Management of finances	7.3	17.2	46.0	23.4

[a]This item was not asked in the DIPO study.

in all tasks, except for those—finances, care organization and transportation—upon which the family seems to want to continue keeping control.

Impact of migrant care work on the role played by the family

A way to understand how the caring role of the family changes as a consequence of the employment of a MCW is to analyse whether, and to what extent, the family network is withdrawing from the provision of some specific care tasks and/or possibly refocusing on different ones. The EUROFAMCARE database allows this analysis, by distinguishing the tasks performed by the primary caregiver (i.e. the family member who is mostly involved in the care of the dependent older person) from the help provided by other family members (Table 2). This information can be further distinguished in order to take into account whether a MCW has been employed and, in this case, whether he/she is living in or not with the cared-for dependent older person.

These findings show that, first of all, when no MCW is employed (cfr. columns 1–3), providing company, care organisation, shopping and transportation represent the main tasks accomplished by the primary family carer (who perform them in about/over 90% of cases). However, while the first two tasks remain in the hands of the primary carers even when a MCW is hired (no matter whether living in or not), shopping and transportation are more likely to be delegated to the MCW (the first more frequently to a live-in MCW, the second more to a non-live-in one). Managing finances and housework are taken upon by primary family carers in four out of five cases when no MCW is present, but the second activity is to a large extent 'outsourced' to the latter as soon as the family opts to acquire his/her help, keeping for itself the control over finances (or even increasing it, in case of a live-in

Table 2 Care tasks performed by (primary and non primary) family carers of dependent older people, by type of support received by migrant care workers (%)[a]

	Eurofamcare						Dipo	
	Primary carer			Other (non primary) family carers			Family carers	
	No MCW	Non-live in MCW[b]	Live-in MCW[b]	No MCW	Non-live in MCW[c]	Live-in MCW[c]	Non-live in MCW	Live-in MCW
	n = 850	n = 35	n = 87	n = 620	n = 24	n = 51	n = 83	n = 137
Care task	1	2	3	4	5	6	7	8
Company	97.3	−0.2	+0.4	86.1	−11.1	−1.8	20.5	10.2
Care organisation	94.0	−5.4	−3.2	48.8	−7.1	−9.6		
Shopping	92.7	−9.8	−13.4	60.7	−5.9	−11.7	15.7	15.3
Transportation	88.1	−13.8	−7.6	56.1	−18.6	−5.1	9.6	16.8
Management of finances	82.2	−5.1	+5.2	48.1	+10.3	−1.0	16.9	25.5
Housework	80.2	−28.8	−34.2	51.9	−1.9	−31.9	4.8	2.2
Medicines administration	75.9	−10.2	−16.1	49.9	+8.4	−20.5	12.0	7.3
Meals preparation/ administration	75.2	+1.9	−22.9	45.9	+4.1	−10.6	6.0	8.0
Lifting/moving at home	74.6	−14.6	−13.7	52.2	−2.2	−18.8	3.6	0.7
Personal care	72.8	+4.3	−14.2	47.1	+7.1	−19.6	3.6	5.8

[a]Figures in **bold** are over 4% above the reference category; *underlined* figures are over 6% below the reference category; *double underlined* figures are over/about 20% below the reference category.
[b]% change compared to the case in which no MCW at all is employed (column 1).
[c]% change compared to the case in which no MCW at all is employed (column 4).

condition). The live-in status of the MCW is decisive for the more frequent delegation of two further activities, meals preparation and personal care, while medicine administration and lifting/moving the older person at home are quite often performed by non-live-in MCWs, too.

A second set of findings emerging from Table 2 (columns 4–6) concerns the other (non-primary) family carers, whose presence in everyday support is in general—compared to the primary carer—much lower for all activities except for providing company. What we can observe in this case is that the impact of the employment of a MCW on the role played by secondary family carers is much stronger (i.e. producing a lower involvement) in the case of a live-in solution, with three exceptions: care organisation, providing company, and especially transportation (from which secondary carers withdraw already or even stronger when the MCW is not living in). The most relevant findings in this respect are, however, that for several activities the presence of secondary family carers increases when a MCW is employed on a non-live-in basis. The EUROFAMCARE findings are partially confirmed by the results emerging from the DIPO study (columns 7–8), highlighting however two main differences: a more frequent provision of company by secondary carers in case of non-live-in MCW; and a higher involvement of secondary carers in managing finances in case of live-in situations.

Impact of migrant care work on the support provided by formal care services

A further aspect which the two studies allow us to investigate is whether the presence of a MCW has an impact on the support provided by professional care services (Table 3). Within the EUROFAMCARE sample, a total of 171 respondents (i.e. 17.3%) reported that professional support was received by the older person in form of care services provided by a public or private organisation (i.e. excluding any form of volunteer work). When no MCW is employed (cfr. column 1), these care services concerned mainly personal care (59%) and housework (42%) as well as—but to a lesser extent—meal preparation and/or administration, help in moving/lifting at home, medicine administration and company.

Once a MCW is privately hired to provide support as a non-live-in home helper (cfr. column 2), the provision of professional support for personal care, meal preparation and housework (i.e. of those types of help which are most frequently delivered by formal care services) decreases to a perceptible extent. Tasks which imply a less intensive hands-on care—such as, for instance, medicine administration, company, transportation, care organisation—seem instead to be more frequently provided.

An even more dramatic drop in the professional delivery of most tasks occurs when a live-in MCW is employed by the dependent older person's family (cfr. column 3), to the point that some types of formal care (such as, for instance, company)

Table 3 Tasks performed by professional care services to support dependent older people, by type of support provided by migrant care workers (%)

	Eurofamcare			Dipo	
	No MCW	Non-live-in MCW[a]	Live-in MCW[a]	Non-live-in MCW	Live-in MCW
	$n = 145$	$n = 11$	$n = 15$	$n = 14$	$n = 7$
Care task	1	2	3	4	5
Personal care	58.6	−13.1	+1.4	28.6	14.3
Housework	41.7	−5.3	−15.0	14.3	0.0
Meals preparation/ administration	37.5	−10.2	−24.2	21.4	0.0
Lifting/moving at home	36.8	−0.4	−16.8	28.6	0.0
Medicines administration	34.7	+10.8	−14.7	21.4	0.0
Company	31.9	+13.6	−31.9	14.3	14.3
Transportation	20.8	+6.5	+12.5	28.6	14.3
Shopping	16.0	+2.2	−9.3	14.3	28.6
Care organization	9.7	+8.5	−3.0		
Management of finances	2.8	+6.3	−2.8	35.7	28.6

[a]% change compared to the case in which no MCW at all is employed (column 1).

'disappear' completely from the list of reported helps. The only two activities which keep on being delivered to a remarkable extent by professional organisations are personal care and transportation. A possible explanation for this could be that care recipients hiring live-in MCWs are usually more dependent (i.e. require round-the-clock supervision) than those who hire non-live-in MCWs, so that severely dependent older people would need a more specialised support (i.e. through professional personal care and transportation by ad hoc equipped vehicles).

While the low number of cases available for these two dimensions (referring to the households employing a live-in as well as a non-live-in MCW and at the same time receiving professional care) invite us to use the above observations with caution, the even lower number of cases in a similar situation emerging from the DIPO database allow us only to confirm at a very general level that, indeed, the live-in option seems to represent a situation likely to induce a sort of crowding-out (replacement) effect of professional care services through the MCW in the field of elder care.

Factors affecting the carer's decision to employ a migrant care worker

In order to better contextualise the above findings, a logistic regression was performed to identify the main factors affecting the family carer's decision to employ a MCW (Table 4).

The findings show that the more severe the disability affecting the older person, the higher the probability that the primary family carer opts for hiring a MCW to receive support in granting the necessary care. Living close to (but not with) the cared-for older person is a further factor directly affecting the carer's decision, as it is his/her employment status, working family carers being twice as likely to resort to the help of a MCW than non-employed carers. A further, interesting observation is that this step is undertaken with a similarly higher frequency by carers who consider as the 'most important' service characteristic the fact that 'care workers treat the older person with dignity and respect'.

Sustainability of migrant care work

A final step in the analysis presented here focuses on the MCWs' willingness to continue being involved in this kind of job as well as on their expectations concerning the future length of stay in Italy. Data show that only a minority of MCWs, even if regularly employed, would like to continue working in this field on a full-time basis (Figure 2), while the majority of them, especially if not regularly employed, had not yet decided whether to settle in Italy or rather to return home (Figure 3).

Discussion

The findings emerging from the two illustrated studies show that the private employment of MCWs by families of dependent older people in Italy has been relieving them from the most burdensome care activities, especially in case of a live-in

Table 4 Factors affecting the family carer's decision of employing a migrant care worker $(n = 892)^a$

Variable name	Categories	Odds ratio	Standard error	Z	P > z
Dependency degree of older person	*Independent*				
	Slightly dependent	1.131	0.966	0.14	0.886
	Moderately dependent	**5.688**	**4.401**	**2.25**	**0.025**
	Severely dependent	**30.922**	**23.540**	**4.51**	**0.000**
Carer's gender	*Male*				
	Female	0.476	0.218	−1.62	0.104
Carer's marital status	*Married/cohabiting*				
	Widowed, divorced/ separated, single	1.519	0.457	1.39	0.165
Kin relationship to elder	*Daughter*				
	Son	0.678	0.388	−0.68	0.497
	Daughter in law	1.340	0.584	0.67	0.502
	Spouse/partner	1.387	0.709	0.64	0.523
	Other	0.789	0.283	−0.66	0.508
Carer/elder place of residence	*Same household*				
	Same building/within walking distance	**3.134**	**1.155**	**3.10**	**0.002**
	Drive/bus, train	1.999	0.807	1.71	0.086
Are you currently employed?	*No*				
	Yes	**2.148**	**0.815**	**2.01**	**0.044**
Good relationship with elder	*Often*				
	Sometimes	0.633	0.373	−0.78	0.438
	Always	1.444	0.414	1.28	0.200
Average number of hours of care provided to elder per week		0.994	0.003	−1.70	0.090
How long have you been caring for the elder?		1.000	0.002	0.03	0.980
Support network in care	*Easily*				
	with some difficulties	0.885	0.237	−0.46	0.648
	No	1.338	0.449	0.87	0.385
Type of support considered as 'most important'	*Attend care support group*				
	Information about support available	1.650	2.350	0.35	0.725
	Advice about disease of elder	1.006	1.465	0.00	0.997
	Training to develop skills for caring	1.602	2.436	0.31	0.757
	Activities outside caring	2.312	3.627	0.53	0.593
	Holiday break from caring	1.505	2.199	0.28	0.780
	Activities for elder	1.011	1.508	0.01	0.994
	Help with planning for the future care	0.803	1.250	−0.14	0.888
	Combine employment with caregiving	0.828	1.271	−0.12	0.902
	Talk over problems	2.173	3.511	0.48	0.631
	More money for care	3.677	5.274	0.91	0.364

Table 4 (*Continued*)

Variable name	Categories	Odds ratio	Standard error	Z	P > z
	Changes at home environment	0.480	0.722	−0.49	0.626
Service characteristic considered as 'most important'	*Help is available at the time carer needs*				
	Help fits in with the carer's routines	2.646	2.478	1.04	0.299
	Help arrives at the time it is promised	0.742	0.412	−0.54	0.591
	Care workers are skilled	1.248	0.415	0.67	0.504
	Care worker treat elder with respect	**2.295**	**0.710**	**2.68**	**0.007**
	Care worker treat carer with respect	2.003	1.685	0.83	0.409
	Help provided improves elder's quality	0.588	0.297	−1.05	0.293
	Help provided is not too expensive	1.756	1.085	0.91	0.362
	Help is provided by the same care worker	3.385	3.128	1.32	0.187
	Help focuses on needs of both carer and elder	0.399	0.514	−0.71	0.476

[a]Variables in **bold** are statistically significant.

solution. The shifting from families to MCWs of heavier tasks such as housework and personal care, but even of more delicate ones like the administration of medicines; the 'repositioning' of professional care services in restricted care segments such as more sophisticated personal care and transportation; and the refocusing of families'

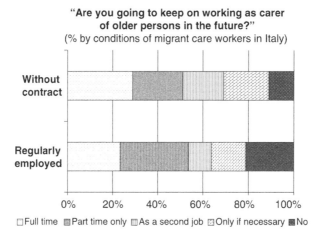

Figure 2 MCWs' answers to the question 'Are you going to keep on working as carer of older persons in the future?', by contractual condition of the MCW.

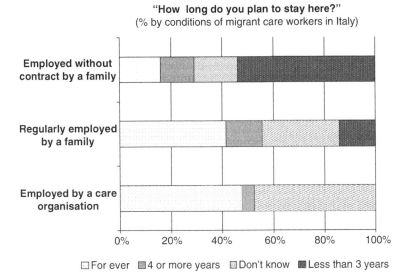

Figure 3 MCWs' plans of staying in Italy, by duration of expected stay.

role on more emotional and organisational activities: these are all elements of an in-depth reshuffling of elder care tasks between old and new actors which has been taking place in Italy in the last few years, at a pace which no one could have expected only a decade ago.

Driven by the matching of an increasing care demand by older people's families, on the one hand, and the supply of cheap care work offered by migrants reaching Italy in an attempt to overcome the poverty affecting their countries of origin, on the other hand, these profound changes occurring in Italian long-term care are challenging the traditional role played by professional services. These are being partly crowded-out by MCWs in most usual care tasks, and are reacting only very slowly to the growing request for more targeted investments and expertise to better train and properly integrate these new actors into the existing formal care network.

The call for a better quality of the care provided by MCWs—a call coming to a large extent also from MCWs themselves (Lamura *et al.*, 2008)—is made even more urgent by the uncertainties concerning the long-term sustainability of the current system, if no new cohorts of MCWs will be found to supplement the current ones, once these will have partly returned back home, or moved to better-paying jobs (in the formal care sector or even in non-care, higher-prestige economic activities) (CeSPI, 2008).

In the light of these challenges, it is crucial to understand which role policies can play, not only at a national but also at a European level, to ensure that this phenomenon occurs in forms that, while respecting the fundamental human rights and interests of all actors involved, can promote a better integration between the privately employed MCWs and the formal care services. This represents not only a widely neglected area of research, but also of reflection by professionals, too, partly also as a consequence of the fact that the employment of most MCWs, despite the reiterated legalisation campaigns, remains largely undeclared in Italy, thus making a systematic dealing with this issue to be considered as unnecessary (MCWs 'don't exist') or superfluous (MCWs 'are not professionals'). The integration between privately paid migrant carers and professional carers represents instead a crucial step to achieve improved care quality standards, by redefining the professionals' role in order to take into account the migrants' presence (Tidoli, 2006).

Elder care policy in Italy—but also in all countries witnessing an increasing employment of MCWs to ensure more care continuity and a more tailored elder care (cfr. Cangiano *et al.*, 2009 for the UK)—is therefore urged to improve the overall quality and attractiveness of the long-term care sector for domestic staff, too. This would, on the one hand, reduce the need to solve current care labour shortages through migration; a practice which, by saving training costs to receiving countries, can however at the same time seriously endanger the low-income sending countries' investments, once their more skilled and enterprising human resources move abroad (Anonymous, 2008), and help to keep in mind, on the other hand, that migrants are not only part of the 'workforce', but also persons, who in the long run might end up becoming, if not adequately protected, one of the population groups more at risk, in terms of health and socio-economic needs, in our society (Watson, 2004).

Notes

[1] This acronym will be used also to abbreviate the term 'migrant care workers(s)' throughout.
[2] These terms will be used as synonyms in this article.
[3] Currently, however, a campaign of over 200,000 controls is being carried out, in order to reduce abuses. First results show that circa 13% of granted allowances might be revoked due to the lack of disability requirements (INAIL, 2009).
[4] For more details on the overall research project refer to the project's homepage: www.uke. uni-hamburg.de/eurofamcare. In-depth information on the survey's sampling and recruitment procedures are reported in Öberg *et al.* (2008).
[5] Details of this study have been previously reported (only in Italian) in Lucchetti *et al.* (2007).

References

Alber, J. & Köhler, U. (2004) *Health and Care in an Enlarged Europe*, European Foundation for the Improvement of Living and Working Conditions, Dublin, Ireland, [Online] Available at: http://www.eurofound.eu.int/pubdocs/2003/107/en/1/ef03107en.pdf (accessed 30 Sept. 2009).

Aliaga, C. & Romans, F. (2006) *The Employment of Seniors in the European Union*, Statistics in Focus, Population and Social Conditions, 15, EUROSTAT, [Online] Available at: http://epp. eurostat.ec.europa.eu/cache/ITY_OFFPUB/KS-NK-06-015/EN/KS-NK-06-015-EN.PDF (accessed 30 Sept. 2009).

Anderson, B. (2007) 'A very private business: exploring the demand for migrant domestic workers', *European Journal of Women's Studies*, vol. 14, pp. 247–264.

Anonymous (2008) 'Finding solutions to the human resources for health crisis', *Lancet*, vol. 371, p. 623.

Brown, C. V. & Braun, K. L. (2008) 'Globalisation, women's migration, and the long-term care workforce', *The Gerontologist*, vol. 48, no. 1, pp. 16–24.

Cangiano, A., Shutes, I., Spencer, S. & Leeson, G. (2009) *Migrant Care Workers in Ageing Societies: Research Findings in the United Kingdom. Executive Summary*, COMPAS, Oxford.

CENSIS (2009) *Una famiglia italiana su dieci è badante-dipendente*, Roma, [Online] Available at: http://www.censis.it/ (accessed 30 Sept. 2009).

CeSPI (2008) *Lavoro di cura e internazionalizzazione del welfare: scenari transnazionali del welfare del futuro*, Roma, [Online] Available at: http://www.cespi.it/Delphi-welfare/executive%20 summary%202round.pdf (accessed 30 Sept. 2009).

DIP (Deutsche Institut für angewandte Pflegeforschung e. V.) (2009) *Situation und Bedarfe von Familien mit mittel- und osteuropäischen Haushaltshilfen*, Cologne, [Online] Available at: http://www.caritas.de/aspe_shared/download.asp?id=C82A7BA8CAE60DD9051220FAADA0 8CD8942B018ED9B45B33103FEBC8CF5A052A3AFCBD314328A6E81BB9955530EBF9EC& Description=Projektbericht%20Mittel-%20und%20osteurop%E4ische%20Haushaltshilfen% 20bei%20pflegenden%20Famili (accessed 30 Sept. 2009).

European Commission (2005) *Policy Plan on Legal Migration*, SEC[2005]1680, Communication from the Commission, Brussels, [Online] Available at: http://eur-lex.europa.eu/LexUriServ/ site/en/com/2005/com2005_0669en01.pdf (accessed 30 Sept. 2009).

European Communities (2008) *Employment in Europe 2008*, Office for Official Publications of the European Communities, Luxembourg, [Online] Available at: http://ec.europa.eu/social/ main.jsp?catId=119&langId=en (accessed 30 Sept. 2009).

Eurostat (2007a) *Europe in Figures. Eurostat Yearbook 2006–2007*, Office for Official Publications of the European Communities, Luxembourg.

Eurostat (2007b) *Employment Rate in the EU27 Rose to 64.4% in 2007*, News Release n. 102, [Online] Available at: http://epp.eurostat.ec.europa.eu/pls/portal/docs/PAGE/PGP_PRD_ CAT_PREREL/PGE_CAT_PREREL_YEAR_2007/PGE_CAT_PREREL_YEAR_2007_MONTH_ 07/3-20072007-EN-AP.PDF (accessed 30 Sept. 2009).

Friedman, T. L. (2005) *The World Is Flat: A Brief History of the Twenty-First Century*, Farrar, Straus, and Giroux, New York.

Gori, C. & Casanova, G. (2009) 'I servizi domiciliari', in *L'assistenza agli anziani non autosufficienti in Italia-Rapporto 2009*, ed. Network Non Autosufficienza, Santarcangelo di Romagna, Maggioli Editore, pp. 35–52, [Online] Available at: http://www.maggioli.it/rna/pdf/rapporto 2009-assistenza_anziani.pdf (accessed 30 Sept. 2009).

Holzer, H. J. (2003) *Can Work Experience Programs Work for Welfare Recipients? Welfare Reform and Beyond*, Brief No. 24, The Brookings Institution, Washington, DC.

Iecovich, E. (2009) 'Migrant live in homecare workers in Israel: findings from a recent study', paper presented at the *World Congress of Gerontology*, Paris, 5–9 July.

INAIL (2009) *INPS: revocato oltre il 13% dei sussidi economici di invalidità civile*, Superabile, Contact Center Integrato per la disabilità, [Online] Available at: http://www.superabile.it/ web/it/CANALI_TEMATICI/Salute/Il_Punto/info1391232813.html (accessed 30 Sept. 2009).

INE (2008) *Work Permits Granted to Foreign Nationals for Domestic Work – 1999 and 2006*, Madrid, [Online] Available at: http://www.ine.es/jaxi/tabla.do (accessed 30 Sept. 2009).

INPS (1992) *Banca dati dell' osservatorio sui lavoratori domestici*, Roma, [Online] Available at: http:// www.inps.it (accessed 30 Sept. 2009).

INPS-Caritas/Migrantes (2004) *Immigrazione e collaborazione domestica. I dati del cambiamento*, Roma, [Online] Available at: http://www.inps.it/news/RICERCA_INPS_LAVORO_DOMESTICO_ IMMIGRATO.pdf (accessed 30 Sept. 2009).

ISTAT (2008) *Rilevazione sulle forze di lavoro. Serie storiche trimestrali 2004–2007*, Rome, [Online] Available at: http://www.istat.it/salastampa/comunicati/in_calendario/forzelav/20080320_00/ (accessed 30 Sept. 2009).

Kaska, S. (2006) *The New International Migration and Migrant Women in Turkey: The Case of The Moldovan Domestic Workers*, MiReKoc Research Projects 2005–2006.

Kavounidi T. (2004) *Survey on the Economy and Social Integration of Immigrants*, PAEP Studies, Athens, [Online] Available at: http://www.paep.org.gr/gr/mod/fileman/files/erevna.pdf (accessed 30 Sept. 2009).

Lamura, G., Melchiorre, M. G., Principi, A. & Lucchetti, M. (2008) *Migrant Workers in the Eldercare Sector: The Italian Experience*, Retraite et Société, Selection 2008, Caisse Nationale d'Assurance Vieillesse, Paris.

Lamura, G., Melchiorre, M. G., Quattrini, S., Mengani, M. & Alberini, A. (2001) 'Chapter 5: Italy', in *Family Care of Older People in Europe*, ed. I. Philp, IOS Press, Amsterdam, pp. 97–133.

Lamura, G. & Principi, A. (2009) 'I trasferimenti monetari', in *L'assistenza agli anziani non autosufficienti in Italia-Rapporto 2009*, ed. Network Non Autosufficienza, Santarcangelo di Romagna, Maggioli Editore, pp. 69–82, [Online] Available at: http://www.maggioli.it/rna/pdf/rapporto2009-assistenza_anziani.pdf (accessed 30 Sept. 2009).

Lethbridge, J. (2007) 'Changing care services and labour markets', paper presented at the *EPSU Social Services* seminar, Athens, 10–12 June.

Lucchetti, M., Socci, M., Gattaceca, R. & Mazzoni, E. (2007) *Donne straniere nel lavoro di cura ed assistenza agli anziani*, INRCA, Ancona.

Ministero della Salute (2000–2007) *Rapporto annuale sull'attività di ricovero ospedaliero*, [Online] Available at: http://www.ministerosalute.it/programmazione/sdo/sdo.jsp (accessed 30 Sept. 2009).

Öberg, B., Quattrini, S., Brown, J., Lüdecke, D., Prouskas, C. & Synak, B. (2008) 'Sampling, recruitment and representativeness', in *Family Carers of Older People in Europe–A Six-Country Comparative Study*, eds G. Lamura, H. Döhner & C. Kofahl, Lit Verlag, Hamburg, pp. 75–116.

OECD (2005) *OECD in Figures. Statistics in the Member Countries*, OECD Observer, Paris.

Pesaresi, F. & Brizioli, E. (2009) 'I servizi residenziali', in *L'assistenza agli anziani non autosufficienti in Italia-Rapporto 2009*, ed. Network Non Autosufficienza, Santarcangelo di Romagna, Maggioli Editore, pp. 53–68, [Online] Available at: http://www.maggioli.it/rna/pdf/rapporto2009-assistenza_anziani.pdf (accessed 30 Sept. 2009).

Redfoot, D. L. & Houser, A. N. (2005) *We Shall Travel On: Quality of Care, Economic Development, and the International Migration of Long-Term Care Workers*, AARP Public Policy Institute, Washington, DC, [Online] Available from: http://assets.aarp.org/rgcenter/il/2005_14_intl_ltc.pdf (accessed 30 Sept. 2009).

Schneider, U. & Trukeschitz, B. (2008) *Changing Long-Term Care Needs in Ageing Societies: Austria's Policy Responses*, University of Economics and Business, Vienna, [Online] Available at: http://cis.ier.hit-u.ac.jp/Japanese/society/conference090114hosei/Paper_UlrikeSchneider.pdf (accessed 30 Sept. 2009).

Suter, B. (2008) *The Different Perception of Migration from Eastern Europe to Turkey: The Case of Moldovan and Bulgarian Domestic Workers*, [Online] Available at: http://aa.ecn.cz/img_upload/6334c0c7298d6b396d213ccd19be5999/BSuter_MigrationfromEasternEuropetoTurkey.pdf (accessed 30 Sept. 2009).

Tidoli, R. (2006) 'Le metamorfosi dell'assistenza domiciliare', *Prospettive Sociali e Sanitarie*, vol. 2, pp. 6–10.

Timonen, V., Convery, J. & Cahill, S. (2006) 'Care revolutions in the making? A comparison of cash-for-care programmes in four European countries', *Ageing and Society*, vol. 26, no. 3, pp. 455–474.

Tinti, V. (2004) 'Sistema RUG: risultati della prima rilevazione', paper presented at the conference '*Il sistema RUG*' (The RUG system), Agenzia Sanitaria Regione Marche, Ancona, 6 Feb.

UN (2006) *Population Ageing Chart 2006*, UN Department of Economic and Social Affairs, Population Division, New York, [Online] Available at: http://www.un.org/esa/population/publications/ageing/ageing2006chart.pdf (accessed 30 Sept. 2009).

US Census Bureau (2008) *International Data Base. Midyear Population by Age and Sex. Projections for 2008 (Table 094)*, Washington, DC, [Online] Available at: http://www.census.gov/cgi-bin/ipc/idbagg (accessed 30 Sept. 2009).

Van Bastelaer, A. & Blöndal, L. (2003) *Labour Reserve: People Outside the Labour Force*, Statistics in Focus, Population and Social Conditions, 14, EUROSTAT, [Online] Available at: http://www.eds-destatis.de/en/downloads/sif/nk_03_14.pdf (accessed 30 Sept. 2009).

Watson, K. (2004) *Minority Elderly Health and Social Care in Europe*, PRIAE Research Briefing. PRIAE, Leeds, [Online] Available at: http://www.priae.org/docs/MEC%20European%20Summary%20Findings2.pdf (accessed 30 Sept. 2009).

WHO (2006) '*Working Together for Health*', The World Health Report 2006, WHO, Geneva, [Online] Available at: http://www.who.int/whr/2006/whr06_en.pdf (accessed 30 Sept. 2009).

Migrant workers in eldercare in Israel: social and legal aspects

Esther Iecovich & Israel Doron

Most old people want to remain in their homes and age in place, and they regard institutional admission as a last resort. In various developed countries, as the demand for homecare workers to augment traditional family caregiving increases apace, migrant caregivers providing otherwise unavailable informal services are becoming more common. They enable older people to stay in their homes, provide them with a sense of security and confidence, reduce feelings of loneliness and solitude, alleviate the family burden, and improve the well-being of the primary caregivers. On the other hand, migrant caregivers pose serious challenges to existing social and legal institutions in the societies in which they operate. They demand policy responses that in many cases have socio-economic consequences that go beyond the older population they serve.

This article describes and analyzes the Israeli experience with migrant homecare workers for older persons. It discusses key problems and dilemmas that are involved with employing migrant homecare workers, and provides some critical perspectives on policies adopted in Israel as a response to this phenomenon.

Introduction

Israel is a young country that was established only 60 years ago, with about 7 million citizens. Despite its young age, Israel is a rapidly aging society with older people currently composing 10% of its population; this is expected to increase to 15.3% by 2025. The age-group of 75+ represents 46.2% of the total elderly population (Brodsky *et al.*, 2009). However, the 80+ age-group is expected to grow significantly between 2007 and 2050, more than any other age-groups (US Census Bureau, 2008; Brodsky *et al.*, 2009). Israel is also among those Western countries with the highest life expectancy. Life expectancy in Israel is 79 for men, 82 for women, and 81 overall (World Health Organization, 2008), which is quite similar to that in some Western European countries such as Austria and Germany. Life expectancy is projected to increase to 81.38 by 2015 and 82.27 by 2025 (US Census Bureau, 2008), which equates to an increase of one year each decade.

Since advanced age is connected with higher rates of morbidity and disability, the proportion of those aged persons who are frail, either physically or cognitively, and need assistance with activities of daily living (ADL) is estimated to be about 16.5% of those aged 65 and over, with more women than men being disabled (19.8% and 12%, respectively). Among those aged 80 and over, the rate of older persons who need assistance with a least one ADL reaches 39% (Brodsky et al., 2009).

Concurrent with these demographic processes, many changes took place in family structures and roles that limited the ability of the family to meet the growing care needs of its older family members (Iecovich, 2007): (1) the constant decrease in fertility has created smaller nuclear families and this trend is expected to increase. For example, currently the number of children per woman in Israel is 2.9 and is projected to decrease to 2.0 in 2025 (Israel Central Bureau of Statistics, 2007); (2) rates of divorce are increasing, thus creating more single parent families; (3) more and more women join the work force and develop their own professional careers; (4) due to long life expectancy the structure of the family is becoming more vertical, creating families with two generations of older people, with the second generation being more preoccupied with its own ageing and less available or capable of providing care to their parents who are in their 90s or older and who have multiple needs for care; and (5) globalization has brought with it higher rates of migration among younger families who seek better work opportunities and better life conditions, thus leaving their aging parents behind.

The meaning and implications of all these social and demographic changes are a decreased number of potential family caregivers to provide care to their older family members whose care needs are permanently increasing. To meet the growing needs, various countries such as Germany, Japan, the Netherlands, Austria, and Israel (Evers, 1998; Schmid & Borowski, 2000; Ikegami et al., 2003; Theobald, 2009) have enacted legislation that is aimed at assuring home-based supportive services to disabled older persons through the provision of either in-cash benefits or in-kind services. In Israel, those who are frail and entitled (based on income tests) to receive homecare services can only receive in-kind services through registered homecare agencies. However, since the early 1990s, a growing proportion of the frail older population in Israel has employed migrant live-in homecare workers who are supposed to provide care around the clock. This relatively new social phenomenon has posed several key challenges to existing social policies, generating public debates and controversies (Kemp & Raijman, 2008).

In light of this background, the goals of this paper are three-fold: First, to describe the development of homecare services that are provided by migrant workers in Israel; second, to discuss the social and legal aspects of employing migrant live-in homecare workers and examine the roles that are played by social workers in this context; and third, to address some key issues that relate to the employment of migrant live-in homecare workers.

Migrant workers in elder care—an overview

According to the push-pull theory on migration (Lee, 1966), people move from one country to another mainly because of social and economic conditions in the place of destination that impelled or encouraged them to do so. This is also true for migrant workers in elder care who leave their families behind and look after older people because of a shortage of manpower in the destination countries whose population is rapidly aging. Poverty and the inability to earn enough or produce enough to support oneself or a family in the home country are major reasons behind the movement of work-seekers from one country to another. Yet, the work that migrant workers do is usually poorly paid and of low status, so citizens are happy to pass this on to migrant workers (Browne & Braun, 2008).

Estimates say that nearly one in six people in the world, which means more than one billion people, cross national borders as migrant workers. Of these one billion, 72% are women (Department for International Development, 2007). However, migration politics in many Western countries towards migrant workers in general and migrant workers in elder care in particular are not integrative. The effect of these policies is usually the marginalization of migrant workers, which takes the form of low incomes, unskilled jobs, and abuse. Some of these issues with regard to migrant homecare workers in Israel will be addressed later.

As noted above, one concern is how to meet the growing needs of frail older persons who live alone or without easily available family members to care for them. One strategy that is becoming more common in various developed countries, such as the United Kingdom, Austria, Sweden, Italy, the United States, Canada, and Israel, is to hire live-in caregivers from abroad, who compensate for unavailable informal caregivers by providing homemaking services and personal care (Redfoot & Houser, 2005).

The issue of migrant live-in homecare workers has been insufficiently addressed in the gerontological literature, in spite of the increase in many Western countries of older persons being cared for by such persons, either legally or illegally. In Italy, for example, it is estimated that about 50% of homecare workers are migrant nationals (Polverini & Lamura, 2004). This reliance on migrant workers is likely to grow in an era of globalization that is characterized by an influx of migrants from developing countries to developed countries in search of work to sustain families left behind. Most of the migrant workers will come from countries such as the Philippines, India, China, Mexico, and the nations of sub-Saharan Africa, the Caribbean, Eastern Europe, and the Pacific Islands (AARP, 2005).

Migration of migrant homecare workers is part of a larger global phenomenon that includes health workers (e.g., nurses, nurses' aides, midwives) who provide care in hospitals and long-term care facilities. However, there is a growing unmet demand for health workers in high-income countries due in part to rapidly aging populations, resulting in more professional agencies actively sourcing workers internationally (WHO, 2006). Although the family remains the most important caregiver and is expected to continue to be so, the use of live-in migrant homecare workers is also expected to expand. Van der Geest *et al.* (2004) provide several examples in which the involvement of a stranger in the care of a parent was regarded as a respectable and appropriate solution for the problem of absent children and grandchildren, provided there was good quality of care.

In most cases, the elderly person lives alone with the paid caregiver. In Italy and in Greece, for example, most of those with migrant homecare workers are severely dependent; in particular, mentally frail (Rothgang & Lamura, 2005). Also, in Austria and Germany mainly older adults with severe care needs are cared for by migrant workers on a 24-hour basis, primarily in middle class families that are able to cover the cost of this service (Theobald, 2009). These homecare workers are considered to be an irreplaceable support for older persons and their families. Their presence around-the-clock helps to significantly decrease the family's burden and allows many families to work and lead normal lives while continuing to provide some care for their elderly members, thus filling the traditional role played by family caregivers (Polverini & Lamura, 2004).

The development of homecare services provided by migrant workers

Since the mid-1980s, 'aging in place' has become a core component in the policy on aging in Israel. Based on this policy, the 'Long-Term Care Insurance Law' was enacted in 1986, and its major aims were two-fold: First, to enable frail older people to age in place; and second, to sustain, support, and encourage family caregivers to assume responsibility for their elderly family members. In this framework, homecare workers are supposed to fill the gap between the elder's needs and the family's care. Essentially, they perform tasks that in the past were performed by the family.

To meet these growing needs for homecare services, to cope with the shortage of indigenous homecare workers who are not willing to do these jobs, and to help the aging population avoid institutionalization, the Israeli government has decided to allow the recruitment of migrant live-in homecare workers to fill these gaps. These workers are supposed to co-reside with the older persons and provide care around the clock (Iecovich, 2007). Thus, during the early 1990s homecare agencies started to recruit migrant live-in homecare workers.

The massive recruitment of migrant homecare workers was part of a broader transition of the Israeli society from a socialist-collective oriented society to a more neo-liberal and individualistic society (Ram, 2005). This political transition, influenced by broader global neo-liberal forces, resulted in a general policy of the government to privatize social services, a trend that started in Israel in the early 1980s. According to this policy, the primary responsibility for caring for frail elderly people lies with the family, thus releasing the State from spending more national resources on institutional care, which is much more expensive than community care. Furthermore, this new policy was further legitimized and institutionalized when, in 1991, the Law of Foreign Workers was enacted, which will be addressed later.

From an historical perspective, Kemp and Raijman (2008, p. 105) describe three main stages in the Israeli policy towards migrant workers: The first stage, 1993–1996, was characterized by 'open skies', i.e., uncontrolled free-market growth of legal permits for migrant workers: from fewer than 10,000 permits in 1993, to almost 106,000 permits in 1996. The second stage, 1996–2001, was characterized by sobriety. Widely publicized stories of harsh exploitation of migrant workers by unscrupulous employers, along with a growing trend of migrant workers to become de facto residents, marrying and having children in Israel, forced a public outcry for government intervention. The government indeed reacted: various economic and legal instruments were developed in order to supervise and regulate this rapidly developing labor market. This stage culminated in 2000, when significant amendments were made to the Foreign Workers Act, providing fundamental employment rights to migrant workers and equaling their employment rights to the minimum employment rights under Israeli law. The final stage, since 2001, is characterized by governmental attempts to 'close the skies', i.e., significantly reduce the number of migrant workers' permits and expel illegal and de facto foreign migrant workers. A strong example of this new policy is the establishment in 2002 of a new police force: the 'Immigration Police', whose duty is to locate and expel illegal migrant workers as well as to punish employers and companies who hire illegal migrant workers. Indeed, in its first two years of operation, 118,105 migrant workers left Israel, of which about 40,000 left under a court order executed by the new police (Kemp & Raijman, 2008, p. 136).

To date, there are about 57,000 migrant live-in homecare workers in Israel, of whom about 47,000 provide care to about a third of the total frail older persons living in the community in Israel. In the beginning, most of them came from the Philippines. Later on, workers were recruited from Eastern European countries such as Russia, Ukraine, Moldova, Romania, Bulgaria, Poland, and recently from Nepal, India, and Sri Lanka (since some Eastern European countries joined the European Union, there are very few workers coming from Romania, Bulgaria, and Poland because they prefer working in neighboring European countries). These formal caregivers are employed by the care recipients; almost all of them co-reside with the care recipients and provide care around the clock. This suggests that, for the most part, the migrant worker shares her or his life with the care recipient and sometimes substitutes for family members who are unavailable.

Policies toward migrant workers in Israel

There has been an ongoing debate in Israel about the appropriate policies that should be adopted with regard to the employment of migrant workers.[1] There are some explicit policies pertaining to various aspects of recruitment, employment, and supervision of legal migrant workers, and there are also rules pertaining to the deportation of those who are illegal and punishment of those who employ illegal workers. However, there are still unclear policies with regard to the absorption and integration of migrant workers into Israeli society. These relatively new policies have been expressed in a series of new laws, regulations, and administrative rules that have been enacted since 1991 as well as amendments to various older laws. There are three major laws that relate to migrant workers in general, including migrant homecare workers:

(1) The Law of Foreign Workers was enacted in 1991 and since then has been amended several times. The law was followed by various regulations and rules. The law prohibits the employment of illegal migrant workers, and details the requirements and the circumstances under which migrant workers can be employed. To avoid abuse and exploitation the law also defines the rights and obligations of migrant workers, including their wages and fringe benefits, such as: appropriate dwelling conditions, health insurance, and holidays, and also establishes that a written contract should be signed between the employer and the migrant worker in his or her mother tongue.

(2) The Law of Employment through Private Workforce Agencies: This law was enacted in 1996 and determines that migrant homecare workers should be recruited only through licensed agencies that must meet some licensing requirements, including guidelines on how migrant workers should be recruited and employed. New regulations that came into effect in January 2009 determine that specific agencies for migrant homecare workers will be established and legally registered, and that these agencies are obliged to run training programs for the homecare workers in their home countries. Also, these agencies have to employ social workers who are supposed to supervise their work and make sure that both sides are getting along, an issue that will be addressed more specifically later.

(3) The Law of Entrance to Israel, which was amended (Amendment no. 9) in 2001. The law states that to become a legal migrant worker one needs a work permit and a visa. Those who do not have these two documents are liable to be deported from the country.

An important factor in the formation of Israel's policies towards the migrant worker population was the third sector, and the NGO community. Since migrant workers started to arrive in Israel in the early 1990s, several non-governmental advocacy organizations were established whose purposes are to protect and promote the rights of migrant workers (*Kav-LaOved*—Workers Hotline; Physicians for Human

Rights; Hotline for Migrant Workers; Association of Civil Rights in Israel). These organizations have been playing a very significant role in promoting the policies towards migrant workers and their legal rights, such as the Health Order of Migrant Workers that was enacted in 2001, which enables them to receive a wide range of health care services. These organizations help them to petition the courts and even the Supreme Court in cases of exploitation, abuse, or violation of rights. There are some court decisions—discussed later—that helped to improve the employment conditions of migrant workers and are actually legal precedents that relate to all migrant live-in homecare workers. There is also a permanent parliamentary committee on migrant workers that addresses various problems relating to migrant workers and initiates new legislation as well as amendments of existing laws and regulations to accommodate them to the changing reality. As some researchers argue, NGOs were actually the leading force in compelling both the local and central governments in Israel to regulate and provide fundamental rights for the migrant worker community (Arkin & Arkin, 2004).

Social workers' roles in homecare services to frail elders

As noted, to enable elderly people to age in place, the long-term care insurance law was enacted. The law defines several roles that social workers should perform. The long-term care insurance law determines that local committees should include social workers from the municipal welfare department, nurses from primary health clinics, and representatives of the national insurance institute. These local committees, which for the most part are headed by social workers, are in charge of determining the package of services that will be provided to those who are entitled to receive the long-term care benefits and of determining the service suppliers from amongst a list of approved suppliers. The package that can be supplied under this law include: homecare services, daycare centers, alarm systems, diapers to those who are incontinent, and laundry services. Further, according to the national insurance institute regulations, agencies that supply homecare services must employ professional workers that include social workers, nurses, and gerontologists. The duties of these professional workers are threefold: (1) to recruit and assign a suitable homecare worker to the care recipient; (2) to monitor the services that are provided to the care recipient and intervene whenever there are problems, including changing of the homecare worker. For this purpose the professional worker has to conduct home visits to the care recipient at least once every two months, and stay in contact with the care recipient, the primary caregiver, or the homecare worker; (3) to run training programs for the homecare workers in order to equip them with basic knowledge on aging processes and interpersonal communication skills. These regulations relate, however, to all the homecare workers that are employed by a homecare agency, including migrant homecare workers.

However, new regulations that came into effect in January 2009 relate specifically to migrant homecare workers that are recruited through manpower agencies.

According to these new regulations these agencies have to employ social workers whose duties are: (1) to conduct home visits to the elderly persons in order to diagnose their needs prior to the assignment of a suitable migrant homecare worker and to examine the conditions that are offered to the migrant homecare worker at the care recipient's home; (2) to conduct a second home visit during the first month after the assignment of the worker, and talk with the care recipient (or family) and with the worker to make sure they get along; (3) conduct home visits at least once every three months. In these home visits the social worker has to supervise the care provided by the worker, provide information to the care recipient's family about the rights of the worker, resolve specific problems, and provide information to the homecare worker about his or her rights and to whom to apply when they are violated; (4) prepare home visit reports and every three months prepare a periodic report that relates to all the home visits and their findings; and (5) to report to the person in charge about any exceptional events such as sexual harassment or abuse of the worker as well as maltreatment or abuse of the care recipient by the homecare worker, including involvement of the police when this is necessary. In other words, the new regulations assign a key role to social workers in supervising the quality of care provided to the care recipients by migrant homecare workers, and in protecting the rights of the migrant workers. The real test will be the extent to which this will work and be enforced.

Key issues

Although there are specific laws and regulations that are supposed to regulate the recruitment and employment of migrant workers, there are still key issues that Israeli society is handling today regarding its social policies toward migrant workers in the field of elder care. We will not attempt to cover all of these issues, but rather present some key issues that, in our view, are representative and of relevance to other societies that are facing similar challenges:

Marginalized ethnic groups

There are no comprehensive governmental policies with regard to the status of migrant workers. Generally, migrant workers who come from the same country or same continent establish social networks and community systems that later become ethnic minorities. To date, in Israel there are three major ethnic minorities of migrant workers: Filipinos, Latin Americans, and Africans. These minorities have established their own community services that are aimed at providing the daily needs of their members such as churches, social clubs, and kindergartens. Although most of them are concentrated in central regions of the country, they become marginalized ethnic groups in the Israeli society (Kemp & Raijman, 2008). Further, many of the legal workers become illegal workers at some point (when they leave their employer or when their visa or work permit expires and they don't renew it), exposing them to arrest and deportation or further abuse and exploitation.

In addition, there are no national policies relating to the criteria that entitle an elderly person to employ a migrant live-in homecare worker. Consequently there are currently no policies with regard to the maximum number of work permits that are provided to migrant homecare workers in elder care. Only very recently, the finance minister appointed an inter-ministerial committee to examine the criteria of entitlement to receive work permits with the intention to significantly reduce the number of migrant homecare workers, so that only those who have very severe care needs will be allowed to employ migrant live-in homecare workers.

Evolution of the grey care market

'Importing' migrant workers in the field of elder care is a huge profit-making industry. The workers pay an enormous amount of money even before they enter Israel to manpower companies and brokers. These brokers, both in Israel and in the country of origin, are responsible for finding an older person in Israel who is entitled to personal care, and for all the authorizations to legally enter and work according to Israeli law. The brokerage companies earn millions and thus have a significant economic incentive to bring more and more foreign workers to Israel (Livnat, 2006; Kav-Laoved, 2008).

Since most of the money is made through brokerage, it is not surprising that the companies lose interest in the migrant worker once he or she has entered Israel and paid the brokerage fee. Indeed, in recent years many stories have surfaced regarding migrant workers who paid enormous amounts of money in order to work in Israel, only to find out once they arrived that they had fallen for a fraudulent scheme: their legal status was not taken care of, and they very quickly faced deportation due to lack of a valid work permit (Rita Lagra *v.* Ministry of Interior, 2006).

This reality has intensified due to a legal policy that was known for many years as the 'binding policy'. Under this legal scheme, a migrant worker had an 'individualized' working permit, i.e., could work only caring for a specific older person. Once that older person died, moved to an institution, or simply fired the migrant worker—situations that in some cases occurred after a very short period of employment—the worker automatically lost his or her work permit and was required to leave Israel. This legal policy turned very quickly into a social backlash. The brokerage companies abandoned the migrant workers, as they had already received the brokerage money, and their future profit was to come from the brokerage of new workers, not from finding a new job for the existing ones. The migrant worker, on the other hand, had no choice but to illegally find another job in order to cover the costs she or he had already paid to enter Israel. The outcome was that in a relatively short period of time an *informal economy* of migrant workers evolved in Israel. According to one report, between 2003 and 2006 the number of foreign workers that entered Israel was four times larger than the number of legal permits issued during that period of time (Sinai, 2006). Naturally, these illegal workers were exposed to exploitation and abuse, as any complaint to the courts or the police would result in their deportation.

Abuse and exploitation

There are many cases of exploitation and abuse on both sides. During the past two years the mass media have reported cases of elderly persons who were abused by their live-in homecare workers. The most tragic case happened a year ago when a Moldovan homecare worker murdered an elderly woman she was taking care of and later committed suicide in prison. When she was arrested, she claimed that the care recipient made her crazy because she did not pay her what she should and was too demanding. There are also many other cases of emotional, physical, and financial abuse, in particular in cases when the care recipient is mentally frail. It should be noted that most migrant homecare workers are women, suggesting that on one hand this role is perceived as low rank but on the other it is perceived as a role in which love and care toward the care recipient are involved. Caring for mentally frail or severely physically disabled elderly people entails hard work around the clock, resulting in emotional and physical burnout. Furthermore, since the migrant homecare workers are far from their families and their natural social networks, seldom can they afford to travel to their own countries for holidays because of the high expense. Thus, they become fictive kin of the care recipients with whom they develop some kind of intimacy and family-like relationships (Karner, 1998; Piercy, 2000). This in turn can impose pressure on the migrant homecare worker to perform more and irregular tasks as well as to work more hours because of the close and emotional relationships that develop between them. Further, because they become fictive kin, they feel uncomfortable refusing to perform certain tasks or to leave their employer on whom they are dependent. To this one should add the significant ethnic and cultural differences of the care recipients and care providers. Most migrant homecare workers come to Israel from countries with different cultural and religious backgrounds and speak different languages. Specifically, most of the migrant homecare workers in Israel are from the Far East, particularly the Philippines; they are Christians, and speak either their national language or English, whereas most of the care recipients are Jewish, most of them speak Hebrew, and were born in European or Arab countries. These cultural differences can create communication problems, verbal and nonverbal alike, that can be frustrating to both sides. These conditions can result in abuse and violence against the helpless care recipients. Yet, it should be emphasized that these cases are rare and most migrant homecare workers are very devoted to their care recipients. However, no research has been conducted in this field and therefore very little is known about this problem.

There are also many cases of migrant homecare workers who are being sexually harassed or abused by either the care recipients or their adult children (Kav-Laoved, 2008). Since these workers are dependent on their employers, many of them are afraid to complain, although there are voluntary organizations to which they can apply for help and protection. They can also apply to the agency that recruited them in their country and ask to work in another place. But there are many cases in which one day the worker just leaves his or her employer and looks for other jobs, thus becoming an illegal worker.

The gap between law on the books and law in reality

As described above, throughout the years, various legal instruments and regulations were established in order to accommodate fundamental rights for migrant workers in Israel. Legal schemes such as mandating the payment of minimum wage, providing health insurance, placing limits on brokerage fees, or mandating the providence of minimal human accommodation are all examples of such protective legal policies.

Still, a significant gap exists between the rights accorded to migrant workers on the books, and the rights they actually enjoy in their daily experience. For example, in 1998, Israel's State Comptroller reported that the majority of migrant workers received wages that were below the legal minimum wage (Office of State Comptroller, 1998). To date, after many legal amendments and reforms to minimize the gap and to ensure basic occupational rights to migrant workers, the gap persists. For example, Kav-Laoved, an Israeli NGO that specializes in the rights of migrant workers, reported in 2008 that in reality the enforcement of labor laws and rights for migrant workers is insufficient, and many of them do not enjoy the minimal rights they deserve (Kav-Laoved, 2008).

Should working hours laws apply to home-based nursing care?

The legal difficulties surrounding migrant workers do not only relate to the enforceability of existing rights. There are also other serious issues that relate to what rights they should enjoy. As discussed above, during the early years of the phenomenon, no specific legal regulation existed in the field of migrant workers, and the result was that in reality the general labor laws did not apply. Only in the second stage, after enacting and amending the Foreign Workers Act, did migrant workers enjoy similar general labor law rights that exist under Israeli law and applied to every worker. Nevertheless, several legal issues remained unresolved.

One such issue was the question of whether Israel's Work and Rest Hours Act (enacted in 1951) is applicable in the field of homecare. In general, under Israeli law, the 'standard' working day is 8 hours of work. If the working day exceeds this framework, then the employer has the duty to pay overtime (which is a significantly higher hourly rate). However, the act itself recognizes types of occupations and positions that are exempt from this general rule. One such exemption exists in cases where the conditions and circumstances of the work cannot supervise or make a distinction between work and rest. The question that was raised is whether migrant workers, who live 24 hours a day in the homes of the elderly persons, and provide care around the clock, are entitled to overtime or should receive a global payment only. The most important case in this field was the Johana Tudoranjan case (2002), brought before Israel's National Labor Court. The court's majority decided that in light of the nature and work-pattern of homecare, one cannot effectively distinguish between times of work and times of rest, hence, global payment was proper, and there was no duty to pay overtime. Nevertheless, in order to compensate for the potentially long hours of work, the majority ruled that an additional 30% compensation should be added to the minimal salary. Two judges dissented, and argued that it is not a proper socio-legal policy to exclude the homecare industry outside the scope of the universal protective labor rights legislation, and that de facto one can distinguish between work and rest, even in this sphere of occupation.

While this decision still stands, the public debate in this field continues in Israel, as NGOs in the field continue to battle for the recognition of migrant workers' right to receive overtime when providing 24 hours of home care. On the other hand, elderly rights organizations in Israel have made the argument that, in reality, the majority of older persons in need of homecare cannot afford to pay overtime, and thus, if such a policy would be adopted, many of them would need to move into institutions, and lose their right to 'age in place'.

Time limits for work permits in the field of elder care

Another example of the difficulty in setting a simple and rational legal policy in the field of elder care provided by migrant workers is in setting time limits for the stay in Israel. In order to prevent the 'transformation' of migrant workers into de facto residents of Israel, various regulations limited the duration of the working permit to a maximum of five years. While this policy seems rational in theory, in the practice of elder care, it created significant humanitarian dilemmas. Take, for example, the case of Hana Martinowski (2006), a migrant worker from the Philippines caring for a 75-year-old Holocaust survivor. The elderly woman suffered from Parkinson's disease and from a mental illness (depression). A very close and intimate relationship developed between the older woman and her carer. However, in light of the fact that the migrant worker exceeded the five-year term, the Ministry of the Interior asked the worker to leave Israel. The older woman's family turned to the court, and pointed to the extreme mental and physical implications for their mother if she had to break the ties she developed with her homecare worker. The court accepted this argument and, based on humanitarian considerations, ordered that the migrant worker be allowed to continue her caring work. As stated by the court's decision (p. 6):

> The State of Israel cannot turn its back to an older citizen, a Holocaust survivor, suffering from mental and physical illnesses, by strictly implementing the rules of law, once there is a real danger of life threatening deterioration of the physical and mental status of the older person.

This court decision is only one example of a general judicial policy that has evolved in Israel in recent years in the field of migrant homecare workers. Over the years, the courts in Israel have adopted a liberal policy toward migrant workers in the field of elder care, while mirroring an understanding of the unique needs of both the older population and its caring population. For example, see the following statement from the Rita Lagra case (2006, p. 3):

> The importation of migrant workers has come to serve needy frail elderly in Israel. This need is more significant than in other occupational fields such as construction, and the legal policy should be more relaxed and flexible. The Ministry of Interior in this field should not only place in front of its eyes the strict implementation of the words of the law, but also the harsh burden faced by the older citizen as a result of such an implementation.

Recruitment and training

Finally, it should be noted that migrant homecare workers are recruited in their home countries without any scrutiny with regard to their mental health and personality. According to the Israeli regulations, the recruiting agencies have to assure that the recruited workers do not suffer from any severe or contagious diseases. Yet, no information is collected regarding the suitability of the worker to provide care to helpless and handicapped people. It should be noted that recent rules published in Israel require the recruiting agencies to assure suitability of the recruited worker to meet the needs of the elderly person, but no guidelines were provided regarding how to meet these requirements.

Further, most live-in homecare workers come to Israel without any preparation or formal training that equips them with caregiving skills and knowledge about coping with various problems that are connected to caregiving, in particular when the care recipient is mentally frail. Although there are some countries, such as the Philippines and Nepal, where specific schools were established to train homecare workers for 'export' and they get some basic training on elder care and the culture of the country where they are supposed to work, this is only a drop in the ocean and most migrant homecare workers come with no training or previous experience. To this, one should add the different cultural habits and codes, and language barriers that in some cases cause verbal and non-verbal communication problems. During the past few years, specific training programs have been run specifically for migrant live-in homecare workers, but these are very limited. Lack of communication, knowledge, and skills expose some care recipients to mistreatment or abuse. The new regulations mentioned above determine that agencies that recruit migrant homecare workers should develop training programs in the sending countries so that when the homecare workers arrive in Israel they are already equipped with some caregiving skills and knowledge. The future will tell us to what extent these requirements are really enforced and implemented.

Conclusions

Migrant workers in elder care in Israel are becoming a significant factor in enabling frail elderly people to age in place and avoid or delay institutionalization. Yet, this issue is entailed with various problems that should be addressed. Social workers have to play a core role in addressing these problems:

(1) They have to become more familiar with and aware of the various laws and regulations, and their complexity, relating to migrant homecare workers' rights and obligations in order to minimize cases of abuse and exploitation on the part of the migrant homecare workers.

(2) Migrant workers are a vulnerable group of people who are dependent on their employers and are hardly cognizant and knowledgeable about their rights, which can be easily violated. Thus, social workers who are more familiar with the various legal aspects of the employment of migrant workers can also empower them by providing them with vital information about their rights and thus prevent or reduce cases of rights violation.

(3) Social workers have to play an active role in intervention in cases of conflicting relationships between the homecare workers and their employers, in particular around issues that relate to the clarification of tasks that homecare workers should or should not perform and the division of labor between the family carers and the migrant live-in workers.

(4) Taking into account the cultural differences and the communication difficulties between the migrant homecare workers and their employers, social workers can serve as facilitators who can help both sides to overcome communication barriers and better understand each other.

(5) In sum, the issue of migrant workers in elder care is a challenging one in all areas: policy, practice, and research. Although it is rapidly becoming a global issue, in particular in many Western European countries, there is a lack of empirical and systematic knowledge about the issues addressed in this paper. Therefore, more research can provide evidence-based professional tools and better intervention methods to social workers and help them to better address the various problems that are connected with this field of elder care.

Note

[1] Migrant workers in Israel are allowed to be employed only in specific economic fields, which include agriculture, ethnic restaurants, construction, and homecare services.

References

AARP (2005) *AARP International Forum on Long-term Care*, [Online] Available at: www.aarp.org/research/international/events/ltcforum_landing.html (accessed 16 Dec. 2004).
Arkin, K. & Arkin, N. (2004) 'Personal welfare services for foreign workers: a normative analysis of the "central v. local" tension', *Haifa Forum for Social Work*, vol. 2, pp. 15–49.
Brodsky, J., Shnoor, Y. & Be'er, S. (2009) *The Elderly in Israel: Statistical Abstract 2007*, Jerusalem, Brookdale Institute.

Browne, C. V. & Braun, K. L. (2008) 'Globalization, women's migration and the long-term care workforce', *The Gerontologist*, vol. 48, no. 1, pp. 16–24.

Department for International Development (2007) *Moving Out of Poverty—Making Migration Work Better for Poor People*, [Online] Available at: http:/www.afid.gov.uk/Pubs/files/migration-policy.pdf (accessed 15 July 2008).

Evers, A. (1998) 'The new long-term care insurance program in Germany', *Journal of Aging And Social Policy*, vol. 10, no. 1, pp. 77–98.

Hana Martinowski et al. v. The Ministry of Interior (2006) A. A. 1228/2006, Administrative Court in Tel Aviv, Tel Aviv, Israel.

Iecovich, E. (2007) 'Live-in and live-out homecare services and care recipient satisfaction', *Journal of Aging and Social Policy*, vol. 19, no. 4, pp. 105–122.

Ikegami, N., Yamauchi, K. & Yamada, Y. (2003) 'Long term care insurance law in Japan: impact on institutional care facilities', *International Journal of Geriatric Psychiatry*, vol. 18, no. 3, pp. 217–221.

Israel Central Bureau of Statistics (2007) *Statistical Abstract of Israel 58*, [Online] Available at: http://www.c.b.s/gov.il/reader (accessed 17 July 2008).

Johana Tudoranjan v. Tzia Maayan (2002) L.A. 1113/2002, National Labor Court in Jerusalem, Tel Aviv, Israel.

Karner, T.C. (1998) 'Professional caring: homecare workers as fictive kin', *Journal of Aging Studies*, vol. 12, no. 1, pp. 69–82.

Kav-Laoved (2008) *Information Sheet: Income from Illegal Foreign Workers*, Kav-Laoved, Tel-Aviv. (in Hebrew)

Kemp, A. & Raijman, R. (2008) *Migrant and Workers: The Political Economy of Labor Migration in Israel*, Van-Leer 1837/06, Administrative Court in Tel Aviv, Jerusalem.

Lee, E. (1966) 'A theory of migration', *Demography*, vol. 3, pp. 47–57.

Livnat, I. (2006) *Chinese Workers in Israel*, Kav Laovd, Tel-Aviv. (in Hebrew)

Office of State Comptroller (1998) *State Comptroller's Annual Report No. 49*, Government Press, Jerusalem. (in Hebrew)

Piercy, K. W. (2000) 'When it is more than a job: close relationships between health homecare workers and older clients', *Journal of Aging and Health*, vol. 12, no. 3, pp. 362–387.

Polverini, F. & Lamura, G. (2004) *National report on Italy: Labour Supply in Care Services, Ancona: Italy*, Instituto Nazionale di Riposo e Cura Anziani, Department of Gerontological Research, Ancona, Italy.

Ram, U. (2005) *The Globalization of Israel*, Resling, Tel-Aviv.

Redfoot, D. L. & Houser, A. N. (2005) *'We Shall Travel On': Quality of Care, Economic Development, and the International Migration of Long-Term Care Workers: Research Report*, AARP Public Policy Institute, [Online] Available at: http://www.aarp.org/research/longtermcare/quality/inb104_intl_ltc.html (accessed 27 Nov. 2005).

Rita Lagra v. The Ministry of Interior (2006) A.A. 1837/06, Administrative Court in Tel Aviv, Tel Aviv, Israel.

Rothgang, H. & Lamura, G. (2005) 'Labour market participation, income and migrant care workers', paper presented at the *EUROFAMCARE* conference, Brussels, Belgium.

Schmid, H. & Borowski, A. (2000) 'Selected issues in the delivery of homecare services to the elderly a decade after implementing Israel's long-term care insurance law', *Social Security*, vol. 57, pp. 59–81. (in Hebrew)

Sinai, R. (2006) 'The number of nursing workers entering Israel is 4 times the number of permits', *Ha'aretz*, 6 Sept., pp. 272–284. (in Hebrew).

Theobald, H. (2009) 'Restructuring elder care systems in Europe: policy-field, policy transfer and negative integration', paper presented at the *ISA RC 19 Conference 'Social Policies: Local Experiments, Traveling Ideas'*, Montreal, Canada, 20–22 Aug.

US Census Bureau (2008) *International data base (IDB): Country summary – Israel*, [Online] Available at: http://www.census.gov/ipc/www.idb/country (accessed 17 July 2008).

Van der Geest, S., Mul, A. & Vermeulen, H. (2004) 'Linkages between migration and the care of frail older people: observations from Greece, Ghana and The Netherlands', *Ageing and Society*, vol. 24, no. 3, pp. 431–450.

WHO (2006) *The World Health Report 2006—Working Together for Health*, [Online] Available at: www.who.int/entity/whr/2006/en/ (accessed 10 Dec. 2006).

WHO (2008) *World Health Statistics*, [Online] Available at: http://www.who.int/whosis/whostat/ EN_WHS08 (accessed 17 July 2008).

Towards a model of externalisation and denationalisation of care? The role of female migrant care workers for *dependent* older people in Spain

¿Hacia un modelo de externalización y desnacionalización del cuidado? El papel de las mujeres migrantes cuidadoras de personas *dependientes* mayores en España

Belén Agrela Romero

Focusing on the Spanish case, this article aims to contribute to the debate on the transformations affecting the so-called new model of eldercare.[1] It outlines the transition towards a care provision model characterised by externalisation and denationalisation, which means the transference of care tasks to women from outside the family group who are mostly foreign. It draws primarily upon the connection established between the Welfare State, the feminisation of migrations and global care chains. The article notes the limitations of the public system of protection of elders, as well as those of formal care services, making eldercare reliant upon family involvement. Since the high cost of private companies' services cannot be met by all family budgets, resorting to migrant carers emerges as a strategy/solution to the problem. We argue that the conditions in which the equation dependent elders-migrant carers is formulated favor the (re)production of social inequalities related to gender, class and nationality. Consequently, migrant care workers become a new potential 'group' for social work practice.

Centrándolos en el caso de España, este artículo pretende ser una contribución al debate sobre las transformaciones que están modulando el llamado nuevo modelo de cuidados.[2] Exploramos la transición hacia un modelo de provisión de cuidados caracterizado por la externalización y desnacionalización, que refiere a la transferencia de las tareas del cuidado hacia mujeres de fuera del ámbito familiar, quienes son mayoritariamente extranjeras. Dirigiremos en primer lugar nuestra atención sobre las conexiones establecidas entre el Estado de Bienestar, la feminización de las migraciones y las cadenas globales de cuidado. El artículo muestra las limitaciones del sistema público de atención a mayores, así como la de los servicios de cuidado formal, que hacen recaer sobre las propias familias el cuidado de mayores. Dado que el coste económico tan elevado ofrecido por las empresas privadas no puede ser soportado por todos los presupuestos familiares, recurrir a las mujeres inmigrantes cuidadoras emerge como una estrategia/solución para resolver el problema. Planteamos que las condiciones en las que se concibe la ecuación mayores dependientes—mujeres inmigrantes cuidadoras favorecen la (re)producción de las desigualdades sociales de género, clase y nacionalidad. En consecuencia, las mujeres migrantes cuidadoras se han convertido en un potencial 'grupo' de atención en la práctica del trabajo social.

Introduction

Two of the most striking features that characterise present-day Spanish society are the progressive rise in the number of older people, which has led to a generalised ageing of the population, and the sustained process of immigration coming from non-communitarian countries. To some extent, both processes are connected. The increase in the ageing population, progressively more dependent when it comes to performing the activities of daily life (ADL), has entailed a demand for the satisfaction of needs that are not entirely covered by the family or the State and that can not always be defrayed through private services. This has generated an informal market directed toward older people in which foreign women are prominent. The scarcity of public policies and social services that target elders, combined with new family models, care conceptions and, above all, the incorporation of women—the traditional caregivers—into the remunerated labour market, has resulted in the search for new strategies with which to approach eldercare.

Incorporating non-national 'other women' into the domestic environment is an increasingly popular solution. Considered as *natural* (biological) caretakers for dependent people *par excellence*, immigrant women are becoming the main actors. As native women are unwilling to carry out these tasks, the eldercare market has generated a progressive feminisation of migration. Immigration thus becomes a resource to face the deficiencies of a welfare state that does not take the necessary measures to assist its elders (Martínez, 2008). A connection is established between the native *passive* population (beneficiaries of Social Security, potential users of assistance services and mostly care-dependent) and the foreign *active* population (whose members contribute to Social Security and are incorporated into the market as service providers).

The Spanish situation is characterised by a weak welfare state model and strong reliance on the family, mostly on women: sustainers and providers of the tasks of reproduction and care. It has also undergone rapid change in terms of migration: from a country of emigration, it has become a country of immigration. The number of registered foreigners has risen by over 4 million in only 8 years (5,220,577 on 1 January 2008). Compared with the other countries of the OECD, Spain occupies the second position in absolute terms of received immigration, preceded only by the USA (Pajares, 2008).

The objective of this debate article is to analyse the current role of migrant care workers in relation to older dependent people in Spain. We first introduce some notes on contextual factors in order to understand this situation: (1) the rapidly ageing of population of Spain, (2) the lack of formal care (even after the implementation of the new National Law for the Promotion of Personal Autonomy and Dependent Care in 2006; from here on, referred to as Dependency Law), (3) the increasing presence of women in the labour market, which has resulted in (4) a shortage of informal care. These factors have led to a situation in which 'importing' female immigrants has become something of an 'informal solution' among both policy-makers and people who require the services provided by immigrants. To analyse how this point has been reached, we contextualise the old age care system to evidence the deficiencies of the public system and the emergence of the private sector. Then we explore and show how a new care model is being configured characterised by the externalisation and denationalisation of care.

Dependent older people in Spain: general characteristics of the care-provision system

In Spain, aging of the population is one of the demographic features that defines contemporary society. The current rate of growth of the older population in developed countries is more than double that in developing countries, and is also double that of the total world population (Kinsella & He, 2009). Beyond a quantitative perspective, this fact implies important challenges to public policies in general and to social work in particular.

According to the last report on the older population in Spain (Ministry of Health and Social Policies, 2008), the number of people above 65 years of age has risen from 5.2% to 16.7% of the total population. Spain occupies the fifth position among the most aged countries on the planet (United Nations, 2008) and, according to the predictions of the Spanish National Institute of Statistics, this number is expected to reach 29.9% of the total population by the year 2060. It is also characterised by an increase in the number of people who live beyond (and will live beyond) the age of 80. It is the aging of aging, also called the 'fourth age.' The extension of life expectancy does not imply that those who live longer are 'free of disability',[3] and the octogenarian population does not always enjoy good health. Statistics show that this age group suffers the most domestic accidents, 61.7% of population (Institute for Migrations and Social Services [IMSERSO], 2009). Added to this is the fact that this cohort does not always have a family support network, good purchasing power or a wide spectrum of public resources and services to cover its needs (physical, emotional, sanitary). This situation is particularly common among women, who have often not had remunerated jobs or high-salary qualified contracts during their active life. They therefore tend to experience a decline in their living conditions when they become widows as a consequence of the lower income received from the widowhood pensions. This is a risk factor for suffering illness and entering a process of dependency.

The higher proportion of widows, due to their longer life expectancy and the higher male mortality consequent upon the age difference within marriages (IMSERSO, 2009), means that dependent men can rely on the support of their wives to assist them but not vice versa. While 4 out of 5 elderly men are married (79.9%), 1 out of 2 elderly women are widows (44.5%) (IMSERSO, 2009). The figure of the wife-caregiver is therefore much more common.

Strategies adopted for the provision of eldercare are diverse and complex (Agrela, 2010). Depending on their family's situation and composition, their economic level, their place of residence, the public offer of care services, etc., people choose between different solutions, which are frequently combined, resulting in mixed modalities of management and execution. The main alternatives are: the informal support of the family (which is still central, carried out by women); public programmes offered by the State (denominated *by proximity*, with limited coverage); the private market (with high costs, not accessible to all citizens); or the irregular market (of which an important section of immigrants are becoming a part).

The 'cushion' of family-based strategies: the weight falls on women's shoulders

The aging of Spain's population has taken place alongside the political, social and economic changes that have latterly transformed the traditional family model mostly, due to women's emancipation. Starting in the 1960s, the so-called 'silent revolution' has liberated women from many of the duties attributed to the female sex. It has been influenced by factors such as: the lower incidence of moral, traditionally Catholic values, in/regarding women or feelings of obligation/responsibility to the family; women's incorporation into the remunerated labour market outside the home; women's access to higher education and their unwillingness to abandon their jobs to form a family; or the higher geographic dispersion among family members.

These mutations have not been accompanied by a more equitable distribution of housework between men and women (Izquierdo, 2003). According to the Eurostat report (2009) on the distribution of housework, in Spain women dedicate up to 3.5 more hours per day than men to these activities. Most women encounter serious difficulties in reconciling professional work with reproduction 'duties' within the household. With women 'out' of the domestic space, the needs of the aging population, together with those of assistance and care of children, sick people and people with autonomy problems, mean they are faced with the denominated 'care crisis.' Time difficulties in taking care of dependent elders emerge, and this translates into a conflict with care provision.

Policies for the reconciliation of family and work lives have not been efficient (Caixeta *et al.*, 2004): in 2007, 82% of those who applied for leaves of absence to care for dependent persons were women, and, in 2008, this percentage continued to be considerably high (66%), according to the statistics on *re*conciliation presented by the Institute for Women at the Ministry of Equality. Related to care for children, the difference is even more considerable: 94% of the applicants are women (years 2007 and 2008). Regarding the use of time, while women dedicate an average of almost six hours a day to housework, men barely complete two hours and 20 minutes (Institute for Women, 2006). These figures indicate the persistence of traditional gender roles, which are present even in the case of women who have a salaried job outside the home. They confirm that the weight of domestic work, reproduction and care lies mostly on women, resulting in the permanence of the assumption of a double role and a double workday.

At the same time, there has been a transition from strategies that aimed at the institutionalisation of older people in specialised entities such as geriatric homes, asylums, hospitals, etc. to *revised* care strategies that seek to allow elders to stay in their own environment. Since the 1990s, as shown in the last report on older people, public social services offered to keep the elderly person at home tripled between the years 2002 and 2008 (IMSERSO, 2005a, 2009). This policy corresponds to one of the principles set for eldercare: 'the permanence of persons in a situation of dependency, when possible, within the environment in which they develop their life' (Article 3, Dependency Law 39/2006).

Compared to the European context, the promotion of these mechanisms has not, however, translated into an effective implementation of continued home assistance. In view of the absence of public amenities, families have to continue taking care of older relatives at home. This limitation often entails complications when, in addition, a significant proportion of children live far away from their parents, when women (from the family and national) ready to take care of these tasks are scarce, and when retirement (or widowhood) pensions cannot cover the economic expense of a permanent private service for the dependent person.

Despite these data, Spanish families continue to be the main welfare system, the 'cushion' of care for individuals of any age, especially older people in a situation of frailty. Compared to other European countries, the percentage of individuals above 65 years of age who live alone is lower, around 20% (IMSERSO, 2009). In most cases, individuals over 65 live with their descendants or other family members. The number of homes where elders live alone has decreased. Only 1.2% of individuals above 65 live in geriatric residences, although this percentage is higher in the case of women.[4] The connection with the family seems to be more fluid than in other European countries: more than 60% of older Spanish citizens say they have daily contact with their sons and daughters, which is why many older people (72%) care for or are under the care of their grandchildren (IMSERSO, 2009).

All of this reflects the permanence of a living-together model marked by family solidarity. In short, care for older people, which is a social and economic cost, still seems to rest on the shoulders of women (Vega, 2009) following the *family-based model* of the Welfare State characteristic of Southern European countries (Esping-Andersen, 1990; Bazo, 2004).

Provision of social care offered by public social services and private entities

The attention paid to the social protection of older people by Spanish public institutions suffers by comparison to the rest of Europe. Recent advances have occurred without reasonably increasing social protection expenses in the Gross Domestic Product (GDP) (IMSERSO, 2009). According to the EUROSTAT data of June 2008 (cited in IMSERSO, 2009), the specific protection of older people in Spain represents 7.9%, compared to 10.9% of the EU-27; in pensions, 8.9% compared to 12.2% of the EU-27; and in long-term care, 0.3% compared to 0.5% in the EU-27. Similarly, considering the *indicator of effort in social protection* (quotient between social protection expenses and the GDP), Spain is located in an intermediate position (20.8%).[5] In general terms, we may say that Spain's social policies and services are less specialised in protection for elders than those of most members of the EU. It dedicates a higher proportion of its resources to health and unemployment but finances all the other social concepts less, especially family and childhood. This is something that appears as a great paradox when we take into account that the family is precisely the main provider of assistance and care for older people.

From a multilevel model of public organisation, social protection of older people is a responsibility that is decentralized to the level closest to the citizen. Local and provincial governments are those that, through Social Services and the supervision of social workers, offer and manage formal resources. Roughly, two types of care services can be distinguished: (1) *Proximity Services*, which have the purpose of allowing older persons to stay within their own environment, such as: home care service (HCS),[6] tele-assistance[7] and daycare centres,[8] and (2) '*Institutionalised' Resources*, which entail the older person's admission to a centre.[9] Normally, these are geriatric homes or supervised houses distant from their regular place of residence where they receive the appropriate care services depending on their situation of disability.

The financing of social services is structured following the co-responsibility principle: there is a contribution of public funds and a contribution by the beneficiary/user (co-payment), which varies depending on the type of services and the territorial dominion where the services are provided. The coverage index of the HCS (percentage of service users above 65 years of age) is located on average at 4.7.[10] In the case of the tele-assistance service, the coverage index—on average—is 4.72 users for every 100 elderly people. In both, the user profile is clearly female (around 70%). Regarding homes and clubs, beneficiaries who are 65 and older represent 57.29%, while for daycare centres for dependents, the coverage is 0.83%. The importance of the private sector in the administration of centres and available accommodation is significant (59% of the total), although the financing of the services comes predominantly from the public sector. As for institutionalised centres, the coverage of this service is 4.31. As for the financing of the coverage for residential vacancies, 2.2 of every 4.3 are private accommodations, financed at market prices and with an occupancy rate lower than 100%, and the other two are (public and subsidised) accommodations that receive public funding, for which there is high competition within the demand. This means that the distribution of the participation of the public and private sectors in residential services is characterised by a predominance of the private sector both in the management and financing of residential accommodation.[11] In view of these statistics, we can observe that the coverage index has risen only minimally and is still very much below the level of demand.

In 2006, the Dependency Law was implemented. It presupposes the acknowledgement of a right, of a fundamental value, and of a moral and political responsibility in terms of providing care to older (and dependent) people, of covering the needs of those who are in a special situation of vulnerability and who require support to perform the ADL. This law has facilitated the acknowledgement for the first time of the situation of dependency[12] as well as of the subjective rights of these people. This implies the recognition of the non-professional carer's status within the family environment: it contemplates the possibility that, exceptionally, the dependent person may receive economic aid to be assisted by non-professional carers. As shown by the statistics published by the Ministry of Health and Social Policies, the profile of the applicants is mostly female (66%), and a little over half of these women are over 80 years old (51.32%), followed by the 65–79 age range (25.23%).

In practice, the expectations that this ambitious law created have not been met. This is not only due to difficulties connected to financing and to the evaluation processes of the dependency degree[13] (which has varied a lot between the different Autonomous Communities), but also because of the type of benefits admitted: only 63.24% receive financial aid, of which 32.56% are economic grants for the family carer, while 12.53% are destined to provide residential assistance and 6.54% home care. The alternative of the family carer has been favoured over other services. This results in (re)enforcing the role of women in these activities. The law has been criticised by feminists for reproducing the norm of care work as 'women's work' with measures that strive to help women continue caring, in notably precarious conditions (Peterson, 2007, p. 272). No importance is being given to the negative effects entailed by continuing with the axiomatic woman-carer, or to the significance and repercussions that may be implied by offering (almost *symbolic*) economic aid which does not take into account the precariousness in which care labours are fulfilled (Feminist Assembly of Madrid, 2006). These types of measures, which favour women in charge of care duties, are based on the biologisation of the affective dimension required by care and associated with *being* a woman, implying a normative/moral dimension of care that is still not being questioned (rather the opposite). This is the logic that underlies the fact that being a carer continues to be 'a woman thing': the duty of both those who are in and those who are out of the house (Agrela & Langa, 2009).

The private market of institutions which offer social and health services provides a possible solution, although limited only to those who have a higher purchasing power. Together with private residences, home care services represent the most usual forms of care mercantilisation, and those that generate the most employment. The demand for care services is a key factor in the growth of private companies which, contracted directly by the families or subcontracted indirectly by local administrations, offer home care and tele-assistance services.

In Spain, the qualified working class with an average income are excluded from public assistance services because they exceed the established minimum standards that grant access to them. Such families must therefore search for alternative solutions since their income is not high enough for them to afford private care. This is the scenario in which immigrant women are becoming more and more central, replacing non-remunerated family care within the domestic space.

An approach to immigrant workers in the care market for older people

Care and domestic work in private households has become the largest employment sector for migrant women, the majority of whom are undocumented (Gutiérrez, 2007). As has been happening in other countries—for example, in the UK (Cangiano *et al.*, 2009) or Ireland (Yeates, 2009)—immigrant women have emerged as the new social care workforce, as the alternative solution to labour shortages in the care sector. In Spain, their involvement in this kind of labour has intensified since 1998. According to the Survey on Active Population (SAP; National Statistics Institute, 2009a), the incidence of *foreignisation* in this sector is estimated to be almost nine times higher than in others. Considering Social Security registration (up to October 2009), 69.12% of individuals included in the Special Regime of Domestic Service were foreign women. These are the official numbers, but this is a type of work that is in many cases carried out without a contract, inside houses and in an 'invisibilised' way (in every sense). Real numbers are therefore expected to be much higher. Even with a contract, many foreign women contribute to Social Security independently, making their own payments. At the same time, the regulation also favours irregularities since it does not compel the employer to register the employee when less than 20 hours a week are worked. It can be estimated that half of immigrants work in the underground economy (National Statistics Institute, 2009a). This applies in particular to those who work in the home care services: women in an irregular situation who do not have unemployment benefits, and still less severance payments, who fall under the demands of laws on foreigners are in a position of greater vulnerability and are more at risk of facing situations of abuse and exploitation.

One of the most reliable studies carried out by the Ministry of Social Affairs on 'Home Workers. Assistance to Older People' (IMSERSO, 2005b) estimated that, in 2004, 40% of carers hired by households to assist elders were foreigners; a figure that rises to 81.3% in the case of 'live-in' carers. Presently, given the increase in the number of dependent persons and of immigrants in Spain, and considering the limitations of public services, the percentage of immigrant women in charge of the assistance of older people continues to rise.

In spite of the difficulties of approaching this *reality* quantitatively, we may build an approximate profile of the domestic foreign carer. Most of them are Latin-American women, who represent 31% of the foreign population, 60% of whom are women (National Statistics Institute, 2009b). The preference for Latin Americans is directly linked to the social imagination, in which they are seen as better skilled for care tasks, thus creating a specific labour niche for them: they are thought of as sweet, affectionate women, of Catholic origin, sharing a similar culture and the Spanish language, all of which (supposedly) make them ideally suited to be 'servants' (Gil & Agrela, 2008; Agrela, 2009). An employer, interviewed about domestic work in Andalusia in 2009, said:

> I have always had a woman at home to care for my parents. A woman, of course, because, besides cooking, helping them change clothes or taking them for a walk, assisting them requires being patient, treating them well and having a certain sensitivity... And that is a woman thing. I do not expect her to be a nurse or a physiotherapist. Above all, I ask her to treat them as if they were her parents (...). In order to fulfil all of this, I can only have Latin-Americans, who have more skills... the ones that are better qualified for this. Because they are the most similar ones to us, Spanish women, to our culture of affection, of being close to one another, of treating each other lovingly, of showing they matter to you and that you care for them (...). I am telling you the same as my neighbour, my sister or my sister-in-law will tell you. They have other Latin-Americans. All the people I know prefer Latin-Americans without a doubt.

In terms of nationality, Dominicans have traditionally been preferred, followed by Ecuadorians, Bolivians, Colombians or Peruvians, and, to a lesser degree, Brazilians and Argentineans. Filipino people are also notable and are greatly appreciated by the higher classes because of their command of English. In recent years, Rumanian, Bulgarian, Polish or Ukrainian women have started to have a higher presence, and, to a smaller extent, Moroccan women. A study made in Spain by the Ministry of Social Affairs to analyse this question showed that there are many stereotypes associated with nationality: 'to take care of children, Eastern women are best; for the elderly, Latin-Americans, who are more affectionate, but Guineans are better if they need to be strong to move the elder person; if you want her cheap and working long hours, look for an Ecuadorian; and if you want her to work like a dog, then a Moroccan (...); Rumanians have problems giving medication because they do not command the Spanish language, which makes communication with the elderly person difficult' (IMSERSO, 2005a, p. 269). This shows that differences of gender, nationality, class, age, ethnic group, legal status and foreignness underlie the discourses on care and organise both how it is carried out and by whom.

The labour modality is directly connected to the family's preference and to the situation of the dependent older person. Most employers tend to seek great time flexibility for the fulfilment of all sorts of tasks (physical and affective assistance and housework). The *live-in*, or partial *live-in*, modality involves the permanent assistance by the carer, who is 'on call' 24 hours a day to respond to the older person's needs.

The great majority of those who work as 'live-in' assistants are women who have recently arrived in Spain, do not have documentation and work irregularly. Eldercare is a quick way for immigrants to access an income, especially when they are recent arrivals, as they cannot find other jobs. Their personal vital circumstances (they are often alone, with debts resulting from the trip, with a dependent family in their countries of origin) tend to influence their being chosen. In general, once they manage to regularise their situation, have some savings and start to plan the reunification of their family, they change to the 'external' assistant modality (by the hour or full time). There is a higher demand for 'live-in' foreign employees, generally hired under the terms of a submerged economy:

> It's not that I prefer her to be foreign, but it is the only choice. In these conditions, Spanish women no longer want to do this job. Who could you find to be at home 24 hours a day at a 'moderate' price? Private services are terribly expensive, and a Spanish carer is asking me to pay her by the hour, and I can't pay that either. But foreigners, since they need it and many of them do not have family here, are willing to do it. And also, at a cheaper cost, because they do not ask for so much. (...) This way, we are all happy. It's like an exchange where we mutually solve each other's problems. (Female employer, 2009, interviewed in the social service centre)

The assistance to the elder person (bathing, feeding, walking, giving medication, chatting) is usually combined with tasks relevant to household management (cleaning, cooking, ironing, shopping). Over-exploitation often occurs, especially in the case of live-in carers. A recent survey about the time dedicated to care (IMSERSO, 2005b) introduced illustrative data on the diverse types of tasks they perform: almost 100% of caregivers do housework and home management activities, 80% of activities are related to accompaniment (in and outside the home) and a little over 75% of them have jobs related to personal help in the house and to socio-sanitary assistance. They respond to the demand for an 'all-purpose' woman: housekeeper, companion, nurse etc, who should be present when she is needed and out of sight when she is not. An employer told me in a conversation about care in Granada, in 2009: 'Care work involves always being alert and available to know when and what to do, and when one has to leave. Therefore, the job well done is that which solves the needs but is not noticed'. This is an invisible though indispensable labour.

Besides the physical effort that these activities require, carers are required to become emotionally and personally involved with the older person (accompaniment tasks). This is the double 'nature' of care. Families ask for the demonstration of 'good carer' skills, such as affection, sensitivity, and patience. The following advert from a job offer publication in Andalusia, in 2009, provides a very good example of this:

> I'm looking for a responsible Latin-American woman to care for an older person with dementia and difficult mobility. House chores: personal hygiene, cooking, cleaning the house and company. Requirements: kind manners, sensitive and affectionate. 24-hour dedication. Full board and individual room. Two free hours a day and one weekly day off of their choice. 520 euros a month. Urgent. Immediate incorporation.

These character qualities, presupposed because the desired employees are women, are *elusive* merits which are hardly professionally measurable. Amongst other consequences, we would like to bring attention to two matters: (1) dealing with feelings, empathy and affection generated on the part of the carer towards the older person entails a great dilemma when aspects such as the improvement of working conditions or the possibility to change jobs arise; and (2) 'affective requirements' tend to leave carers in a vulnerable position, exposing them to moral or economic blackmail, hours of dedication abuse or justification for hiring and/or firing.

Externalisation and denationalisation of eldercare

The option of resorting to the private market via the (sub)hiring of immigrant women is increasingly popular, with the external carer replacing the family carer. The reconciliation of work and family life is thus solved through the externalisation of care: hiring a woman 'from outside' the domestic unit. Since these women are generally foreign, this externalisation of care combines itself with what has been called the *denationalisation of care* (Castelló, 2008; Agrela & Langa, 2009). Then, care becomes the occupation that allows immigrant women to enter the Spanish labour market (IMSERSO, 2005a), connected to the feminisation of migration. The State and the market are co-responsible for the feminisation of migration flows, responding to a certain national logic which configures the immigration model and profile, but also responding to a certain global logic. Care and domestic work appear as the 'hidden' side of the new economy (Gutiérrez, 2007), (re)enforced by government decisions and migration policies.

The distinctive characteristics of the national informal market in which this activity is carried out are to some extent encouraged by the decisions of government, which organises its migration policies based on the selection of the workforce to carry out activities in certain labour niches which are not covered by Spanish citizens. The invisibility of care, associates to 'cleaning' and 'care giving' activities, gives rise to unregulated and unprotected working conditions (Peterson, 2007; Martínez, 2008). Eldercare activity is ultimately configured under an informal economy which mainly takes place in private spaces that are scarcely inspected in terms of labour conditions and which are favourable to abuses, exploitation, racism, etc. The professionalization of this occupation is constituted under a very fragile and deregularised work regime which promotes irregularity, precarious conditions, low wages and, occasionally, forms of neo-servility and ethno-stratification.

This process of the feminisation of migration connected to care activities also responds to the dynamics of a globalised world and of the new models of economic organisation based on an internationalisation process in Northern and Southern countries.[14] The growing importance of women as starters of migration chains is directly related to changes in the forms of production and reproduction worldwide, which lead, in the countries of origin, to the phenomenon known as 'feminisation of survival' (Sassen, 2002) and, in the contexts of destination, to the demand for a gender-segregated workforce to fulfil certain activities related to care.

Consequently, a great portion of the 'dirty work' (Anderson, 2000) which had so far been taken care of by certain Spanish women has been assigned to immigrants, giving rise to a 'gender specialisation—between men and women and between some women and others—of the nicest (non remunerated) reproductive labours and of the hardest (precarious) labour, which impacts the (affective) management and (physical and emotional) execution of tasks as well' (Caixeta *et al.*, 2004, p. 19). More than half the women who have some sort of care, domestic or cleaning job are foreign, which reveals the ethnisation and feminisation of this new labour niche.

The concept of 'replacement migrations' (UNO, 2000), which establishes a connection between the ageing population and its impact on the feminisation of migrations, linked to the concept of 'world affection chains' or 'global care chains' (Hochschild, 2001), refers to the creation of bonds between women at a transnational level formed with the purpose of sustaining everyday life. The care tasks are transferred from one woman to another based on multiple power factors, amongst which gender, ethnic group, social position and place of origin stand out (Pérez, 2007). So, the globalisation of social reproduction is inextricably linked to economic globalisation (Yeates, 2009): these macro processes have had a direct impact on female international migrations, which should be analysed on the grounds of the inter-connections and inter-dependencies engendered by the global dynamics that generate care chains. Job 'opportunities' for women coming from peripheral countries are therefore created. Women that migrate to assist *our* dependents then find themselves requiring the services of other women in their respective homes of origin to take care of *their* dependents (mostly underage children). These processes provide evidence for the social and economic role of women, both in the productive and in the reproductive sphere, in the societies of origin and destination (Morokvasic, 1993).

Dependent elders, migrant carers: challenges for social work

This article has described an 'emerging social phenomenon' which corresponds to the equation *dependent elders-migrant carers*. Eldercare appears to be a 'provisional solution' both for foreign women and for Spanish families who solve in this way the problem of older people's assistance and avoid the compromises traditionally demanded by women's inequality. This implies the emergence of a new employment source related to proximity services which needs to be deeply analysed by social work, questioning not only the public system's assistance fragilities but also the role assigned to immigrant women as a 'resource themselves'. The normative and ideological framework of migration that makes this possible is being used by the State and the market to (re)enforce the process of *externalisation* and *denationalisation* of care. Care continues to be an invisible, devalued activity, transferred to *other women* who are positioned at the bottom of the stratification chain. The perpetuation of the sexual division of labour (along with divisions of class, race and nationality) implied by the transferring of care and domestic work from one woman to another is hardly being questioned at all. Foreign carers thus embody the paradox of being indispensable people without being wanted, of being inside the nation but not a national citizen, inside the home but outside the family (Macklin, 1999).

The impact of population ageing on the potential future demand for migrant workers in older adult care should be more closely examined at the level of social work and social policy. It is essential to recognise the care work fulfilled by migrants as a growing area of intervention in the Welfare State context (Valtonen, 2001). Social work is much more than a profession which implements policies; from the standpoint of practice we also have to condemn the weight and the way in which public policies legitimate and (re)produce social inequalities related to gender, class and nationality.

Social work is a *hinge* between territories located in the care-related space. It articulates public policies and social proximity services to respond to the needs of families and dependent elders. It is within this field that the degrees of dependency and the resources to be assigned are evaluated. The social worker occupies a space connecting the two parts of the equation: dependent elders and foreign carers. They are in a special position to offer a unique perspective on the deficiencies of a phenomenon that superficially satisfies everybody. Social workers are in a privileged place in the public system. For that reason, they are able to question whether resorting to foreign carers instead of offering public services could be merely an artifice that seeks to hide the cracks and weaknesses of the system of social protection for dependent people.

The consolidation of this feminised and ethnified labour niche buries migrant women under a modality of neo-servility. The presence of migrant care workers opens up many social problems with which social workers will need to engage because they could be a new potential 'group' for social work practice. It suggests the need for the permanent training of social workers to have more empirical and methodological tools to analyse and design efficient social services related to migrant women and elderly people. Raising awareness among the native population is also necessary to highlight the conditions in which the foreign women are living. In conclusion, taking into account their understanding of the social exclusion process, social workers should be more active in questioning the situations and inequalities perpetuated by public policies and advocating a higher level of social justice.

Acknowledgements

The Andalusian Institute for Women, Regional Government of Andalusia, for supporting the research titled 'Family and Migrant Carers. Transformations in the Model of Dependent Care within the New Framework of the Dependency Law' (2009–2010); the G.D. for Migration Policy Coordination of the Ministry of Employment, Regional Government of Andalusia for supporting the research titled 'Immigrant Women in Assistance and Care Services in Jaén' (2010–2011); the European Commission, Seventh Framework Programme for supporting the research titled 'Gender, Migration and Intercultural Interactions in the Mediterranean and South East Europe: an Interdisciplinary Perspective' (GE.M.IC); MICIIN (Ministerio de Ciencia e Innovación) for supporting the research titled 'Migration Policies, Familiar Transnationalism and Civic Stratification. Latinamerican Migration to Spain' I_D_I 2010–2012 (CSO2009-1349) (2010–2012).

Notes

[1] This reflection article is based upon our own research experience in: (1) Research: *'Family and Migrant Carers. Transformations in the Model of Dependent Care within the New Framework of the Dependency Law'*, supported by the Andalusian Institute for Women, Regional Government of Andalusia, (2) Research: *'Immigrant Women in Assistance and Care Services in Jaén'*, supported by the G.D. for Migration Policy Coordination of the Ministry of Employment, Regional Government of Andalusia, (3) Research: *'Gender, Migration and Intercultural Interactions in the Mediterranean and South East Europe: an Interdisciplinary Perspective'* (GE.M.IC), supported by the European Commission, Seventh Framework Programme, (4) Research: 'Migration Policies, Familiar Transnationalism and Civic Stratification. Latinamerican Migration to Spain', MICIIN, I + D + I 2010-2012 (CSO2009-1349).

[2] Este artículo de reflexión está basado en nuestra experiencia de investigación: (1) Investigación: *'Cuidadoras familiares e inmigrantes. Transformaciones en el modelo de cuidados a las/os dependientes ante el nuevo marco de la Ley de Dependencia'*, financiado por el Instituto Andaluz de la Mujer, Junta de Andalucía, (2) Investigación: *'Mujeres inmigrantes en los servicios de atención y cuidado en Jaén'*, financiado por la D.G. de Coordinación de Políticas Migratorias, Junta de Andalucía, (3) Investigación: *'Gender, Migration and Intercultural Interactions in the Mediterranean and South East Europe: an Interdisciplinary Perspective'* (GE.M.IC), financiado por la Comisión Europea, Séptimo Programa Marco, (4) Investigación: 'Políticas migratorias, transnacionalismo familiar y estratificación cívica. Las migraciones latinoamericanas hacia España', MICIIN, I + D + I 2010-2012 (CSO2009-1349) (subprograma SOCI).

[3] The Ministry of Health and Consumer Affairs (2005) uses the term *Esperando de Vida Libre de Incapacidad (EVLI)* (Disability-Adjusted Life Expectancy (DALE)) as an indicator to analyse the Spanish population's health in comparison to the European context.

[4] In Europe, the number of women living in these types of residences is double the number for men. In some countries, like Luxembourg, this ratio is multiplied by three (Iacovou, 2000).

[5]   Very distant from Switzerland's 32%, in the border between the new member countries and the 15 countries which formed the European Union before 1 May 2004. Ten out of the 12 new members are located below Spain's level, together with one of the veterans (Ireland). Two of the most recent partners (Slovakia and Hungary) present higher figures than Spain.

[6]   An individualised programme, of a preventive and rehabilitating character, which articulates a set of services and professional intervention techniques consisting of personal and domestic assistance, psycho-social and family support, and relations with the domestic environment, provided at the dependent older person's house.

[7]   A service that, through the telephone and with computer equipment located in the assistance centre and at the user's home, allows elderly or handicapped people to press a button that they constantly carry with them and to be in verbal contact with professionals who are trained to respond to the urgency.

[8]   Social, sanitary and family support centres that offer assistance during the day for the basic, therapeutic and socio-cultural needs of elderly people with dependency to encourage their autonomy. They are located close to their habitual environments. They are publicly and privately-subsidized. The most common are homes and clubs for the elderly, and daycare centres for dependent elders.

[9]   Residential assistance for the elderly includes the following resources: residential centres, public service of temporary stays and alternative accommodation systems: assisted living facilities, residential apartments or any other resource of residential character (IMSERSO, 2009).

[10] The rise in the number of users has translated into an increase of coverage, which has almost doubled, going from 2.75 in 2002 to 4.69 in 2008.

[11] Eighty percent of residential centres (4,072) are privately owned and they manage 76.7% of residential vacancies (252,712). Twenty-four percent of the residential accommodations (78,828) are run in partnership with the public sector and 53% of them (173,884) are completely private accommodations paid for at market prices.

[12] To access a benefit it is necessary to be evaluated on the degree of dependency by a team of social workers and a medical team. The different types of benefits/services are considered depending on that degree. The situation of dependency is classified in three levels: a) Grade I. *Moderate* dependency: when a person needs help at least once a day to perform their BADL or for intermittent needs; b) Grade II. *Severe* dependency: when a person needs help two or three times a day to perform their BADL but does not want the permanent support of a carer; c) Grade III. *Major* dependency: when a person needs help to perform their BADL several times a day and, due to their loss of physical, mental, intellectual or sensorial autonomy, needs the indispensable and continuous support of another person.

[13] By 1 July 2009, a total of 913,723 applications were submitted, 77.33% of which have the right to be beneficiaries of a service (in the first year, that right was only granted to those who were evaluated as having a Grade III dependency; currently, this is also granted to those with Grade II). Also, differences between the Autonomous Communities have been very important. For example, Andalusia had 231,115 rulings while Madrid had 40,201 (IMSERSO, 2009).

[14] Causes and explanations of women's migrations are to be read in the gender key, 'a factor that may explain not only the feminisation of poverty but female poverty, not only the feminisation of work but female work' (Papí, 2003, p. 57).

References

Agrela, B. & Langa, D. (2009) *Cuidadoras familiares e inmigrantes. Transformaciones en el modelo de cuidados a las/os dependientes ante el nuevo marco de la Ley de Dependencia* [Family and

Immigrant Carers. Transformations in the Model of Dependent Care within the New Framework of the Dependency Law], Women's Institute of Andalusia, Sevilla (2009–2010).

Agrela, B. (2009) 'De los significados de género e inmigración (re)producidos en las políticas sociales y sus consecuencias para la acción e integración social' ['On the meanings of gender and immigration (re)produced in social policies and their consequences for social integration and action'], in *Inmigración y políticas sociales [Immigration and Social Policies]*, eds L. Cachón & M. Laparra, Bellaterra, Barcelona, pp. 239–267.

Agrela, B. (2010) 'Modelos de provisión de cuidados: género, familias y migraciones' ['Models of care provision: gender, families and mgrations]', *Alternativas. Cuadernos de Trabajo Social*, vol. 17, pp. 1–10.

Anderson, B. (2000) *Doing the Dirty Work? The Global Politics of Domestic Labour*, Zed Books, London.

Bazo, M. T. (2004) 'El papel de la familia y los servicios en el mantenimiento de la autonomía de las personas mayores: una perspectiva internacional comparada' ['The role of family and services in sustaining the autonomy of older people: a comparative international perspective'], *Reis*, vol. 105, pp. 43–77.

Caixeta, L., Gutiérrez, E., Tate, S. & Vega, C. (2004) *Hogares, cuidados y fronteras . . . Derechos de las mujeres inmigrantes y conciliación [Homes, Care and Borders . . . Immigrant Women's Rights and Conciliation]*, Traficantes de sueños, Madrid.

Cangiano, A., Shutes, I., Spencer, S. & Leeson, G. (2009) *Migrant Care Workers in Aging Societies: research Findings in the United Kingdom*, Centre on Migration, Policy and Society, Oxford.

Castelló, L. (2008) 'La "desnacionalización" del cuidado y la domesticidad en los Países Mediterráneos. La nueva cara del familismo' ['The "denationalisation" of care and domesticity in Mediterranean countries. The new face of familism'], in *Congress: Los nuevos retos del transnacionalismo en el estudio de las migraciones [The New Challenges of Transnationalism in the Study of Migration]*, Universidad Autónoma de Barcelona, Barcelona.

Esping-Andersen, G. (1990) *The Three Worlds of Welfare Capitalism*, Polity Press, London.

Eurostat (2009) *Harmonised European Time Use Study*, Eurostat, Luxembourg, [Online] Available at: http://epp.eurostat.ec.europa.eu/portal/page/portal/eurostat/home

Ezquerra, S. (2008) *The Regulation of the South-North Transfer of Reproductive Labor: Filipino Women in Spain and the United States*, Dissertation, University of Oregon.

Feminist Assembly of Madrid (2006) 'La ley de dependencia ante la crisis del trabajo de los cuidados' ['The dependency law and the crisis of care work'], *Amaranta*, vol. 2, pp. 1–28.

Gil, A. & Agrela, B. (2008) 'Un mundo en movimiento. Contextualización de las migraciones internacionales en Europa y América Latina' ['A world in motion. Contextualisation of international migrations in Europe and Latin America'], *Revista de Derecho Migratorio y Extranjería*, vol. 19, pp. 263–283.

Gutiérrez, E. (2007) 'The "hidden side" of the new economy. On transnational migration, domestic work, and unprecedented intimacy', *Frontiers: a Journal of Women Studies*, vol. 28, no. 3, pp. 60–83.

Hochschild, A. R. (2001) 'Global care chains and emotional surplus value', in *On the Edge: living with Global Capitalism*, eds W. Hutton & A. Giddens, Oxford University Press, New York, pp. 130–146.

Iacovou, M. (2000) *The Living Arrangements of Elderly Europeans*, ISER Working Paper. 2000-2009, University of Essex.

Institute for Migrations and Social Services (IMSERSO) (2005a) *Cuidado a la dependencia e inmigración [Dependent Care and Immigration]*, Ministry of Labour and Social Affairs, Madrid.

Institute for Migrations and Social Services (IMSERSO) (2005b) *Cuidados a las personas mayores en los hogares españoles. El entorno familiar [Care for Older People in Spanish Homes. The Family Environment]*, Institute for Older Persons and Social Services, Madrid.

Institute for Migrations and Social Services (IMSERSO) (2009) *Las personas mayores en España. Informe 2008* [*Older People in Spain. 2008 Report*], Ministry of Labour and Social Affairs, Madrid.

Izquierdo, M. J. (2003) 'Del sexismo y la mercantilización del cuidado a su socialización: hacia una política democrática del cuidado' ['From sexism and the mercantilisation of care to its socialisation: towards a democratic care policy'], in *Congreso: SARE Cuidar cuesta: costes y beneficios del cuidado* [*Caring Costs: Costs and Benefits of Care*], Emakunde, San Sebastián, pp. 1–30.

Kinsella, K. & He, W. (2009) *An Aging World: 2008. International Population Reports*, U.S. Government Printing Office, Washington.

Macklin, A. (1999) 'Women as migrants. Members in national and global communities', *Canadian Women Studies*, vol. 19, no. 3, pp. 24–31.

Martínez, R. (2008) *Bienestar y cuidados. El oficio del cariño. Mujeres inmigrantes y mayores nativos* [*Welfare and Care. The Trade of Affection. Immigrant Women and Native Elders*], Dissertation, A Coruña University.

Ministry of Health and Consumer Affairs (2005) *La salud de la población española en el contexto europeo y el Sistema Nacional de Salud. Indicadores de Salud* [*Health of the Spanish Population in the European context and the National Health System. Health Indicators*], Ministry of Health and Consumer Affairs, Madrid.

Ministry of Health and Social Policies (2008) *Las personas mayores en España. Informe 2008* [*Older People in Spain. Report 2008*], Ministry of Health and Social Policies, Madrid.

Morokvasic, M. (1993) '"In and out" of the labour market: immigrant and minority women in Europe', *New Community*, vol. 19, no. 3, pp. 459–483.

National Statistics Institute (2009a) *Survey on Active Population*, Madrid, [Online] Available at: http://www.ines.es/jaxi/menu.do?type=pcaxis&path=%2Ft22/e308_mnu&File=inebase&L=O (accessed 2 Dec. 2009).

National Statistics Institute (2009b) *Municipal Register: Foreign Population*, Madrid, [Online] Available at: http://www.ine.es (accessed 1 Dec. 2009).

Pajares, M. (2008) *Inmigración y mercado de trabajo. Informe 2008* (*Immigration and Labour Market. 2008 Report*), Ministry of Labour and Immigration, Madrid.

Papí, N. (2003) 'Clase social, etnia y género: tres enfoques paradigmáticos convergentes' ['Social class, ethnic group and gender: three converging paradigmatic approaches'], *Utopías*, vol. 1, no. 195, pp. 55–75.

Pérez, A. (2007) *Global Care Chains*, Gender, Migration and Development series, Working Paper, 2 UN-INSTRAW.

Peterson, E. (2007) 'The invisible carers: framing domestic work(ers) in gender equality policies in Spain', *European Journal of Women's Studies*, vol. 3, no. 14, pp. 265–280.

Sassen, S. (2002) 'Global cities and survival circuits', in *Global Woman*, eds B. Ehrenreich & A. R. Hochschild, Penguin, London, pp. 42–59.

United Nations (2008) *World Population Prospects: The 2008 Revision Population Database*, [Online] Available at http://esa.un.org/UNPP/ (accessed 1 Aug. 2009).

UNO (2000) *Migraciones de reemplazo: ¿Una solución ante la disminución y el envejecimiento de las poblaciones?* [*Replacement Migrations: A Solution to the Reduction and Aging of Populations?*], Population Division of the UNO, New York.

Valtonen, K. (2001) 'Immigrant integration in the welfare state. Social work's growing arena', *European Journal of Social Work*, vol. 4, no. 3, pp. 247–262.

Vega, C. (2009) *Culturas del cuidado en transición* [*Care cultures in Transition*], UOC Editorial, Barcelona.

Yeates, N. (2009) *Globalizing Care Economies and Migrant Workers: Explorations in Global Care Chains*, Palgrave Macmillan, Basingstoke.

Grandmothers as main caregivers in the context of parental migration

Bunicile ca îngrijitoare in contextul migratiei parintilor

Maria-Carmen Pantea

Whilst a large number of parents from Romania migrate for work, the surrogate-parenting role of grandmothers remains overlooked both in policies and in research. This article explores, through 24 in-depth interviews, the often-invisible experiences of grandmothers, for a more complete understanding of the process of migration and the necessary development of social services. The fieldwork was located in the northern countryside, which has an established culture of migration and in urban and rural areas from Transylvania, where migration is more isolated. Existing policies are mainly aimed at assisting (the often victimised) children 'left behind' and fail to address the needs of the grandmothers. A recent law requiring migrant parents to register a guardian is highly ineffective, as families find their private ways to navigate the process of migration. Grandmothers develop their own coping strategies for managing childcare and for understanding the current process of migration. The article asserts the need for cultural sensitive interventions aimed at increasing grandmothers' individual wellbeing. Their situation has to be contextualised simultaneously in terms of the global dynamic of migration and in terms of the more traditional expectations for reciprocity of care at later age.

In conditiile in care un numar mare de parinti din Romania migreaza pentru munca, rolul de parinte-surogat al bunicilor ramene neglijat atat in politicile sociale, cat si in cercetare. Acest articol exploreza prin 24 interviuri de adancime, experienta adesea invizibila a bunicilor, pentru o intelegere mai completa a procesului de migratie si pentru dezvoltarea serviciilor sociale. Cercetarea a fost desfasurata in zonele rurale din nordul tarii, caracterizate de o cultura inradacinata a migratiei si in zonele urbane si rurale din Transilvania, unde practica migratiei e mai izolata. Politicile existente tind spre asistarea preoponderenta a copiilor, ramasi acasa' si esueaza in a aborda nevoile bunicilor. O lege recenta care solicita parintilor sa inregistreze oficial un tutore este mai curand ineficienta, intrucat familiile gasesc propriile lor cai pentru a traversa procesul migratiei. Bunicile dezvolta strategii de coping proprii, atat pentru cresterea copiilor, cat si pentru a intelege procesul de migratie. Articolul sustine nevoia de interventii sensibile cultural pentru a creste gradul de bunastare al bunicilor. Situatia lor trebuie sa fie contextualiata simultan in termeni de dinamica globala, dar si in ceea ce priveste expectantele traditionale de grija pentru persoanele in varsta.

Introduction

International scholarship has been greatly concerned with incoming migrants. The preoccupation with who is 'left behind' is recent, with a growing interest in children (Pham & Hill, 2008) and in the care provisions following migration (Hochschild, 2000; Parrenas, 2001, 2005; Piperno, 2007). Frequently, grandmothers step in when parents migrate, without much research and policy interest being dedicated to it. This article is exploring the often-invisible experiences of the grandmothers as main caregivers in the context of parental migration from Romania.

Migration from Romania to other European countries occurred gradually: from a male-dominated, mainly illegal migration during the 1990s, to a significant process of male and female migration after 2000. Now an EU member, Romania has a statistically uncertain part of its active population working abroad. Overall, it is estimated that 10% of Romania's adult population has had experience of working in a foreign country at some point after 1989 (Soros Foundation Romania, 2007, cited in UNICEF & AAS, 2008).

The population which migrates to the EU for work is not random. However, there are not enough data to discern their profile. According to Soros Foundation Romania (2007), migrants are mostly from the countryside or small towns, where former industries collapsed, mainly from the north-east region of Moldova (50%). Other regions of Romania involved are the northern and partially south-east. Migration rates decrease further as we go towards the west. It is estimated that 78% of migrant mothers and 63% of fathers are less than 40 years old, with the majority having an average education (UNICEF & AAS, 2008).

The number of the children of migrant parents varies: from the official data of 82,464 (ANPDC, 2007) to estimates of 350,000 (UNICEF & AAS, 2008). According to the last source, 400,000 children experienced the migration of at least one parent, at some point in their life, whereas 126,000 children now have both parents abroad. Moreover, half of them are less than 10 years old, 25% are between 2 and 6 years, and 4% are less than 1 year of age. The percentage of children who spent more than 1 year without both parents is 16%, whereas for those who spent more than 4 years it is 3%. Between 16 and 18% of all children between 11 and 15 years of age have at least a parent working abroad (SFR, 2008). Apparently due to the higher importance of the extended family in the countryside, more than half of the children with both parents abroad are in the rural areas.

Unlike other ethnic groups (including Roma), there does not seem to be a pattern of entire family migration or reunification abroad among ethnic Romanians, even if this is legally possible.[1] Reunification is very recent, isolated and follows a process of successive migration of family members. There are several potential explanations for this: from the increased costs of childrearing abroad, precarious living conditions and occupational demands exerted upon parents (e.g. domestic work of women), to (arguably) adolescents' poor adaptation abroad and perceived education prospects in Romania, the extended family support and, ultimately, poor information on opportunities and benefits in the destination country.[2]

Data on caregivers are scarce: when both parents are migrating, 74% of children remain in the care of grandparents[3] and 5% with other members of the extended family (UNICEF & AAS, 2008). Infrequently, children remain in the care of a neighbor, friend, older sibling[4] or by themselves.

Why do parents migrate? Explaining theories of migration

Internationally, there are several explanatory theories of migration, each having its own shortcomings. According to Phizacklea (1999, cited in Ryan, 2004), the first is the so-called 'push/pull' theory which situates migration in the neoclassical model of rational choice. Given the calculus of economic and social costs/ benefits in country and abroad, migrants decide autonomously. The model was later criticised by the feminist scholarship that argued that families are not unified entities and their members (including children and grandparents) have different positions towards migration (Hondagneu-Sotelo, 1992, cited in Silver, 2006).

Secondly, according to the *household strategy theory* (Phizacklea, 1999, cited in Ryan, 2004; Westwood & Phizacklea, 2001), migration is a means to attain a common plan. The *structural theories* understand migration in its social, economic and political context, shaped by unequal distribution of power and wealth (Westwood & Phizacklea, 2001). This is where one needs to consider Romania's economic context:[5] massive unemployment in the 1990s, regional discrepancies, and reduced prospects for youth, simultaneously with the seduction of a Western consumption model.

A fourth explanation is the *migratory networks* (Westwood & Phizacklea, 2001), instrumental in explaining the large migration flows from several areas and not from others. This is similar with the 'culture of migration' examined by Dreby (2005) in Mexico. It is not always poverty which mobilises migration (Žmegač, 2007). Being rather 'a way of life', than 'a strategy for a purpose', migration becomes part of a shared local culture. Situations of otherwise affluent rural areas of Romania with high migration rates could have such explanations.

More recent research saw migration through the lens of the Western ideology of 'ideal childhood',[6] which motivates parents to migrate and extend their stay indefinitely (Parrenas, 2005; Horton, 2008). In Romania, migration is reinforced by the communist legacy of deprivation and a culture of parental sacrifice (similar with the familial model of sacrifice from Mexico, which in Horton [2008] had a religious explanation). Finally, one should not ignore the demand side of migration. A growing need for domestic work in Western Europe maintains migration from Romania (Piperno, 2007) and reproduces what Hochschild (2000) called 'the global chains of care'.[7] The foreign labour force recruitment mediated by the Romanian government may further legitimise and encourage migration.

Policies and social work services related to migration

Social work with children has long been maybe the most developed sector of social services in Romania. The high international pressure over abandoned children and the risks of institutionalisation have shaped its recent history. Yet, parental migration found Romanian social work services unprepared, and then only following media interest. It is in this context that efforts were focused on the children of migrant parents, with migration being invariably defined as a problem and children, its victims.

The situation of the transnational families entered the policy agenda in 2006, when a Governmental Ordinance had been issued, soliciting parents to inform authorities of their leaving intentions, and register a guardian. Its purposes were manifold: identification of 'children at risk', data collection, awareness rising, service provision and transparent monitoring.

However, the 219/2006 Ordinance soon became ineffective. First, as it applied only to legally migrating parents, the majority of cases remained unreported (Committee on the Rights of the Child [CRC], 2008). It was estimated that as little as 7% of the parents informed authorities about their decision to emigrate (UNICEF & AAS, 2008). The main reasons were parents' concern over their working status in the destination country and the anxiety over a potential involvement of child protection services.

Second, as the Ordinance did not provide standardised actions for assistance, practitioners were left with imprecise guidelines (AAS, 2008; SFR, 2008). As the very definition of 'risk' was interpretable, so were the interventions that followed and which situated social workers at the border of legitimacy. Besides, the Ordinance did not have the compelling regulative power of a law (AAS, 2008).

Given the above limitations, a new regulation was issued in 2009. This was a law obliging migrant parents to nominate a guardian meeting several criteria (a relative with at least the minimum income guaranteed and at least 18 years older than the child to be cared for, full physical and psychological capacity, no disabling conditions or previous parenting convictions, no more than three other children in care). There are substantial fines for parents trespassing the law. Monthly monitoring visits by the social workers, with the ultimate responsibility for child replacement in state care, are stipulated. Even if the law is not aimed at caregivers, it is indirectly protecting grandparents from roles that may potentially harm their health.

Even though Romania has a broad scheme of social assistance provisions (Cerami, 2006, p. 154), older adults seeking age-related services still replicate a more general pattern: in the competition for professional attention and assistance, they are less successful than the younger groups (Monk, 1990; cf. Joslin, 2002). The means tested income-support benefits are administered by local authorities that decide upon eligibility. However, large regional disparities make eligibility conditions variable. Several deprived communities with migrants (especially in the east) have the poorest resources for assistance and interventions.

Bureaucratic demands limit social workers from providing other services. More-over, local authorities may have the assumption that migrant families develop their own internal arrangements and thus, relieve the state of its role (Luca, 2007; UNICEF & AAS, 2008). Overall, existing policies and services that focus on the difficulties encountered by children overlook the needs of elder surrogate parents. The economic crisis (associated with lower remittances) makes necessary interventions even less probable.

Brief description of study

The aim of this article is to bring grandmothers'[8] caring for children of migrant parents[9] from Romania closer to the centre of academic and social concern and, by making their perspectives visible, to contribute to their welfare and empowerment. How are grandmothers embracing the new roles and what are the social expectations exerted upon them? What are the new forms of community that emerge and how are the responsibilities shared between parents, grandparents, children themselves and, ultimately, state institutions?

The research explored, through 24 in-depth individual interviews, the experiences of grandmothers caring for children with migrant parents. The fieldwork was located in Romania's regions of Maramureş and Transylvania, in both urban and rural areas. The research tried to balance the inclusion of accounts from communities with different practices of migration: from an established culture of migration in rural Maramureş and Bistriţa, to villages, towns and cities where migration is rare.

The selection of communities considered the regional differences, which generate different patterns and purposes of migration. Maramureş has rural areas with established networks of migration, not necessarily motivated by poverty (see similar situations reported in Westwood & Phizacklea, 2001; Dreby, 2005; Žmegač, 2007). Transylvania is a region where the migration of both parents is very rare, apparently due to the high urbanisation (UNICEF & AAS, 2008). Implicitly, the social environments surrounding remaining grandparents and children differ: from a community-shared experience of migration (in Maramureş), towards more ambivalent social constructions of the 'atypical' grandparents and children 'left behind' (in Transylvania). For these reasons, inclusion of accounts from different communities was needed.

The identification of informants was a rather difficult process, with intricate barriers. The fieldwork took place in a context dominated by the victimisation of children of migrant parents in media, social work services, NGOs and schools. Portrayed as 'left behind', 'home alone' or 'orphans with parents', their situation was invariably associated with devastating psychological consequences of parental absence (including several child suicides).

Under these circumstances, grandparents' reluctance to share familial experiences was explicable. Without a previous experience of participating in a research, tape recording (although necessary for ensuring the 'trustworthiness' of the data) would have risked causing distress and role confusion. Tape recording would have been associated with journalism and might have installed an imbalanced power relation between the researcher and the interviewed grandmothers. Besides, migration is not a personal, but a familial issue; sharing this experience with a potential stranger means disclosing family matters. For a conservative aged population, this is inappropriate. Also, many grandmothers are occupying an ambivalent position in the family (both in generational and gender terms). They do not entirely act *in loco parentis* and their autonomy is relative, if not even controlled from afar by migrants who may act as gatekeepers for such research.

The process of data collection was inspired by the ethical obligation not to do more harm than good. Interviewing was based on grandparents' informed consent and confidentiality was insured. Twenty-six grandmothers had been approached and two declined/were prevented from participating in the research.[10] They were exclusively approached through close personal contacts. This reduced role confusion and increased trust. The selection bias was minimised by the inclusion of informants with different age, familial, social, economic and ethnic situation.

All interviews (ranging from 30 to 70 minutes) took place in the grandparents' home. Notes were carefully taken (including citations) and reviewed immediately after the interview, while missing data were added. In this way, the collection of data minimised the information lost by the lack of tape recording. In addition, fieldwork was complemented by informal discussions with grandmothers and community members. In the paper, most of the grandmothers' accounts are paraphrased.

Following the research of Mevi-Triano and Paskas in Joslin (2002), the interviews were guided by several general questions: (1) Under what circumstances did grandmothers come to raise their grandchildren? (2) What it is like to be raising a grandchild with migrant parents? (3) How has their caregiving role influenced their own lives? (4) What enables them to cope? and (5) What is their relation with social services? Notes were transcribed and coded successively in Nvivo8. The analysis was based on the main themes that have been generated in relation to the above questions.

Results and analysis

Grandparenting and the culture of mutual obligations

One could not examine grandparenting in the context of migration without an overview of the way the (extended) family is generally understood. Romania has an established culture of dual earner income families. During communism, grandparenting had been a family strategy to cope with childrearing and employment demands, but also with the severe shortage of supplies in the cities. Although nuclear households have long been the norm, some intergenerational connections between rural and urban areas remained.[11] Now, a severely dysfunctional pension system, especially in rural areas, changes the direction of the informal economy and maintains the provision of mutual care in the case of international migration.

Regardless of residence, there is a cultural assumption of parental support long into adulthood and the social expectation that grandparents step in when needs appear (Nesteruk & Marks, 2009). Whereas some involvement of grandparents in childrearing has been a long-standing practice, long-term grandparenting is new. In this context, one could ask, following Gomes' (2007) example of Mexican migration, whether family exchanges are not a substitute for less functional policies (as will be explained later).

The following section explores the perceived lifestyle transformations intervening in grandmothers' lives in the context of migration. The main dimensions that organise grandmothers' caring experience are related to (1) their living arrangements, (2) support networks and (3) relation with existing services. The data analysis is structured along these main dimensions.

Negotiation of living arrangements

Most of the interviewed grandmothers were living in multigenerational households, which appeared to be the rule in the regions with high migration. One could argue that, to some extent, this living arrangement created the enabling circumstances for parental migration in the first place, as it endorses caring expectations towards grandparents.

In rural regions of Maramureş and Bistriţa, the primary marker of migration (and status) is the house, often extremely large, two-storied and opulent. Obviously, the financial support for building and equipping them comes gradually, while migrant parents come and go. Grandchildren's early childhood is simultaneous with the house building. Conversely, in communities with no culture of migration, working abroad is a strategy for overcoming economic impasses[12] and, sometimes, marital discord.

Under these circumstances, grandmothers (mainly in the countryside) embark on simultaneous roles: taking care of the grandchildren (a practice which often continues from their birth), coping with emergent health problems and other nurturing roles. This is the situation of a 63-year-old grandmother from Maramureş village who started demolishing the old house and building a new one with the remote advice from migrant parents. This was at the time her 84-year-old mother passed away, her two granddaughters were 8 and 10 years old and she had to be sympathetic towards a husband with a long-term psychological disorder. The migrant parents came for their first visit in two years, at the time the house was almost ready.

In more vulnerable family situations (e.g. single motherhood, illness), emotional support and increased concern for those abroad may intervene. Mariana,[13] aged 45, a Roma grandmother of two in a suburban village in Transylvania, is afraid for the health of her migrant daughter, with whom she wants to change places as 'a mother is still a mother'. With successive medical interventions following domestic violence, the health of the now single mother raises severe concerns for the remaining grand-mother.

In multigenerational households, being involved in children's school life becomes a predictable extension of the grandparents' role. The pressure exerted by the contact with school is diminished when dissipated among similar others (e.g. grandmothers feel comfortable when there are 'more grandmothers than mothers' at school meetings in a village from Bistriţa).

One leitmotiv in the interviews has been grandmothers' concern for preparing children for school (neat clothing, with cakes for school parties), 'for nobody to guess they have no parents here'. One could argue that this preoccupation with issues that are, ultimately, non-academic, is the only way the working class can respond to children's educational needs (Lareau, 2003). A common strategy for solving school performance problems is *commodification of learning* (grandparents ask about the necessity of paying for extra classroom tutoring).

Previous research shows that mothers' migration rarely destabilises the gendered division of work, as fathers rarely assume the childcare alone. When mothers only migrate, grandmothers are usually undertaking 'women's work' (Parrenas, 2005; Piperno, 2007; Lutz, 2008), often in more precarious economic circumstances and, at times, in the context of family discord. Grandmothers may need to cope with children's contestation of their authority, with father's alcohol consumption, parental divorce, lengthy debates over custody, or highly emotional episodes of departure.

At times, there are outbursts in the negotiation of the tasks, like the discussion between Letitia (a grandmother of two) and Ana (a migrant mother from the neighbourhood, recently back home) demonstrates. Letitia exasperatedly describes her daily work that includes feeding animals, working in the field and preparing lunch for her grandchildren and her son-in-law. She reproaches her daughter's indolence when home and her 'obsession with cleaning the house' (a potential transfer of her domestic work from abroad). When Ana, in a movement of solidarity with Letitia's daughter, tries to justify her attitude by asserting: 'We are coming back so tired that we cannot start it over at home. We work so much there...', Letitia outbursts: 'Yes, right! But we are not working either? We are not tired?' Such disagreements seem to be maintained by migrants' protective tendency to offer pleasant images of their work abroad to their parents. In such a context, frustrations like the one above may be generated.

When a single mother migrates, the economic and social resources available for grandmothers are reduced. Besides, in more cohesive communities, grandmothers need to defend the mothers' choice to migrate, or to balance the risk of desertion. This is the situation of a Roma[14] grandmother from a semi-urban neighbourhood. Her contacts with various institutions have been marked by the anxiety of having one of the boys, with a severe mental disability, placed into state care. With very limited resources available, she made the care of the children a priority.

One should not invariably assume kinship care, or financial aid from migrant parents. For many grandmothers, children's migration continues a life of need and distress. In situations of couple separation, grandmothers develop strategies to cope with family conflict over distance: from the gradual exclusion of an alcoholic father and concentration on providing for the grandchildren, to displays of welfare towards the extended family of the deserting parent.

Yet, in multigenerational households, most grandparents consider their lives would not have been much different, were the parents at home. As in the case of grandparents caring for HIV-infected family members, the above respondents would disagree about calling their tasks 'burdens' as they are simply 'taking care of their own blood' (Schatz, 2007). However, the situation is described relatively differently by grandmothers moving into grandchildren's homes, as presented below.

Grandmothers may leave their own house and join their grandchildren's home (including abroad) for episodes of parental migration. When abroad, the experience is often perceived as alienating (with no knowledge of a foreign language and hesitant about exploring the city): 'I was staying on the balcony as someone on another floor was speaking Romanian. Just to hear . . . or watch a coach going to Romania everyday at 5'. Conversely, for middle-class or educated grandmothers, the concerns related to the situation at home (e.g. husband's poor health), rather than the isolation, make them come back.

When grandchildren remain home, grandmothers may temporarily move into their house (especially in the case of seasonal migration). Over the winter, grandmothers expect to go back to their own home 'to settle down'. Alternatively, 'keeping an eye' on remaining grandchildren, from the grandmothers' own house, is also a practice. When living in close proximity, grandmothers may undertake several errands. Children are also active agents in negotiating the distribution of tasks and, when grown up, they may gradually limit grandmother's involvement. This is the situation of a family where an 18-year-old asked to be registered as a guardian of her younger brother.

Besides the two living arrangements outlined above (continuation of multi-generational living arrangements and grandmothers' relocation to grandchildren's home), a third practice consists of children's relocation to the grandmother's home. The changes in grandmothers' lifestyle are noticeable especially where there has been not much previous contact between the two, or when the experience of bringing up toddlers is remote.

The ways grandmothers incorporate the presence of children in their lives vary. They may develop strategies to accommodate the needs of the children: from providing a space that resembles the one from home, to offering a sense of common ownership by unrestricted access to household and goods. Conversely, grandmothers may impose restrictions over adolescent girls' mobility and social relations or entail work demands.

Grandmothers need to adapt to new situations: from the change of household furniture and commodities (DVD, PC, furniture adjustments), to transformations in family social life. Anastasia, a grandmother from the Transylvanian countryside who had her urban adolescent granddaughters in her care for four years, describes her experience as rejuvenating. She speaks enthusiastically about having the front yard full of teenagers and the door always open, about becoming young peoples' confidant, about gaining the respect of young people in a village that does not value youth cultures.

Conversely, grandmothers may restrict the mobility in the household, a practice that limits children's sense of control and leads to inevitable disagreements: 'I tell them all the time to keep the front room nice and tidy. They are girls'. Occasionally, adolescents' negotiation of power may situate grandmothers in a challenging position. It is in this context that grandmothers may become concerned and refer to migrant parents for mediation. Silvia, an urban grandmother from Transylvania, formerly a teacher, declares herself helpless in dealing with her adolescent grandson's behaviours (e.g. smoking and drinking in the company of some new friends she knows little about). In extreme situations, a granddaughter running away from home may bring increased distress.

Having grandchildren in the same household may take unanticipated forms for grandmothers receiving children brought up abroad. A different language, feeding habits and lifestyle may pose serious challenges. The new family unit has to negotiate its practices, with grandmothers being influential actors in adapting to change and in demanding it.

Networks of support (I): the community of grandmothers

The great majority of interviewed grandmothers did not feel they had considerably changed their habits, or, if they did, they did not experience it as a great loss. In the countryside, children are integrated in the adults' social life to a greater extent than before. As the leisure opportunities for young people in the countryside are very limited, children and grandparents start sharing the same free time activities. Children interfere in the grandmothers' community by inevitably reducing its privacy, a presence experienced as intrusive and objectionable. A new type of neighbourhood emerges: young girls join grandmothers in their Sunday gatherings and gradually, the grandmothers engaged in childcare become unavailable for a customary chat among neighbours.

In addition, the social life of grandmothers is highly dependent on the situation of migrant parents. When their status is problematic (rumours about marital discord and separation, debts), grandmothers tend to avoid social gatherings. By this, they avoid exposing family issues, but also recourse to a potential source of assistance. Informal loans and moral support are available in the situations where a family problem is overt: e.g. a grandmother caring for a child with special needs, irregular remittances, children's abandonment by the remaining father, grandmother's severe illness.

One should not overstate, however, the extent to which the proximity of other grandmothers is of assistance. In the countryside, the privacy of the family is cherished. Sometimes even the minor decisions are taken by consultation with the migrant parents, rather than with the neighbouring grandmothers. On the other hand, when some advice on childcare is shared among grandmothers, it may cause more harm than good: e.g. beating a child to counteract feeding problems, or restricting children's mobility in the household/neighbourhood.

The attitude of the community over grandparenting is ambivalent: from being appreciative ('You are brave. I wouldn't ever dare raising a child of this age'—infant or adolescent) to critical ('I wouldn't give a child so much freedom. Toys everywhere!') or even condemning ('Didn't you raise enough children during your lifetime?'). It is under these circumstances that grandmothers are rather reluctant in sharing significant issues of concern with their immediate community.

In the cities and small towns, grandmothers' attitudes seem different. The immediate community does not exert so much pressure, the situations of grand-mothers as surrogate parents are rare and the incentive to meet women in similar situations (e.g. by a discussion group) higher. To some extent, one could even identify a demand for a social context where issues related to childrearing can be openly discussed. According to grandmothers, the envisioned focus of such meetings would be on childcare techniques and communication strategies with adolescents, and less on the ways of reaching more personal comfort.

Networks of support (II): the extended family

The support from the extended family for the grandmothers is not as unequivocal as one may assume. In the cities, this role is decreasing significantly. Distance, grandparents' reduced mobility, the focus on nuclear family and the simultaneous migration of several family members deprive the ageing grandparents of care and support (Hochschild, 2000; Silver, 2006; Piperno, 2006, 2007; McGuire & Martin, 2007; Lutz, 2008; Pham & Hill, 2008).

In a context of a dysfunctional healthcare system, the traditional practice of family-based care has long been the solution for many elderly persons. However, the *care drain* from Romania and the demographic decline make the provision of services for the elder population one of the most critical issues for the future (Piperno, 2007). Institutions for older people (rare and with extremely long waiting lists) are rather stigmatising options: both for the aged person and for the extended family.

It is under these circumstances that the relation between migration[15] and care becomes ambivalent. On the one hand, migration generates *problems*, as it deprives elderly people of care in terms of domestic work, house maintenance and makes increased demands on their health. On the other hand, it is *a potential solution*, by reinforcing grandparents' expectations for care in older age, and by increasing the possibilities to secure therapeutic interventions and medicines, through remittances.

Whilst in a traditional family dynamic, the expectations of care might have been legitimate, the current changes in family life make grandparents take measures to ensure they will receive the necessary care in old age. One such strategy is the care for grandchildren, not without expectations and moral sanctions attached to their choice. Caring for some grandchildren and not for others is an investment, but it simultaneously diminishes the possibilities to receive old age care from another child.

The research came across situations where grandmothers cared for as many as six grandchildren from three different families. Alternatively, there were situations where a 'selection factor' operated: grandmothers with severe health problems were not caregivers and have been replaced by aunts. Ultimately, few grandmothers declined a caring role, not without a distance being installed between them and the children.[16]

Where care is shared among in-laws, there is also some potential for tension in the extended family, which is ultimately brought to the attention of migrant parents. For the case of babies, at stake are different childrearing practices: lack of stimulation, feeding habits and even charges of physical abuse. Conversely, the removal of a child after a long period of grandparenting may lead to tough adaptation problems, for both the grandparent and the child.

Grandmothers' experiences with the available policies and social work services

Most of the interviewed grandmothers did not have any previous knowledge of social work. Those who did have some contact came from communities with low incidence of migration. Their attitudes towards the social protection services were shaped by the grandmothers' perceived level of control over their situation. At one extreme is the continuous anxiety of a Roma woman, afraid of having a disabled child removed into state care. At the other end is the tranquillity of two middle-class urban grandparents, registered as guardians and who are routinely visited by a social worker who acknowledged that 'everything is fine', but who 'still, has to come'.

Out of the 24 interviewed grandmothers, three were registered as guardians. In rural communities there appears to be some knowledge of the possibility of being documented as guardian, but no grandmother seemed interested in it. They did not experience situations that put them at a disadvantage because of not being registered and the lack of registration was a shared community practice. A formalisation of their status seemed useless.

The attitudes regarding the social provisions provided by the state varied from asserting a reasonable living standard due to their own resources (pension), to the security provided by family arrangements ('I don't need their money'). As the system of accounting for migrants' income is poor, the risk of (arguably) deceptive allocations is present. A potential 'Matthew effect' may, thus, develop: the better informed the grandmothers, the more services/subsidies they manage to reach for themselves or their families (e.g. social aid, free resort ticket, a free computer for children). Conversely, the grandmothers in higher need are also the ones with the poorest information on how to access available resources. This 'Matthew effect' goes along with a practice of claiming benefits from an impersonal state, which may occasionally include the grandmother's speculative strategies of hiding the migration from authorities, with several controversies in a community being generated. Yet, the majority of interviewed grandmothers did not expect and were distrustful of any state-provided assistance.

Concluding remarks

Unlike other EU countries, the history of dealing with migration is very recent in Romania. Mainstream social workers may not recognise the international dimension of the problem or may lack the instruments to do so. There is a tendency of approaching children with migrant parents as being abandoned children, when in fact their situation is, most of the time, fundamentally different. Reading their situation invariably through the lens of child abandonment (as it appears to be the case in media, social work practice and even in several NGO reports) (Piperno, 2006) is severely misleading. It is also a grave injustice done to grandparents and it risks doing more harm than good.

Future legislation need to balance children's rights to assistance, parent's right to free circulation and work and grandmothers' welfare and family's right to private life. The 2009 law on guardianship is welcomed, as it rectifies numerous shortcomings of the previous regulations. A family plan of social assistance is among the policy proposals of the moment. This would be the first measure for financially assisting caregivers of children with migrant parents. While legislation has to be unitary, future services need to be developed in ways that are sensitive to the high regional discrepancies in Romania and in patterns of migration. What may work for one segment of the population may not work for another.

The law's penalty-focused character may be an incentive for some parents, but not the ultimate solution for many. In regions with an established culture of migration, customary family strategies are in place and there will be a need for culturally sensitive campaigns (endorsing family solidarity and parental sacrifice simultaneously with the need to legalise the guardianship). There, the 'bonding social capital' (in-group particularised trust) increases the reliability of the family and decreases the influence of state institutions.

While previous interventions tended to concentrate on children, an added focus on grandparents would be needed. Yet, in a collective understanding of family life, potential interventions need to be sensitive to the fact that in traditional rural areas, elderly focus on individual well-being may be ill placed. During the interviews, grandmothers found it difficult to speak of personal feelings. Under these circumstances, interventions aimed at increasing grandmothers' welfare need to be framed in terms of the family welfare.

Interventions need to be culturally sensitive. Support groups among grandmothers and respite care, for instance, may be valued in the cities, but would not work in the countryside, where family secrecy prevails. Absence of parental care is an awkward issue and social workers risk being perceived as interfering in family life. After precarious media reporting, social work needs to reconstruct its image in ways closer to its social mission.

It becomes evident that grandparent's well-being needs to be understood in the global context of migration. However, when it comes to monitoring situations that reach beyond frontiers, social work in Romania definitely lacks the necessary resources. There is a need for knowledge and skills in cross-country casework (Hendriks *et al.*, 2008), issues that have not been addressed in social workers' training. For the time being, there are poor technical resources for connecting social workers with migrant parents or with other social workers abroad. Romania needs to develop swift information flows with similar services from receiving countries. Similar proposals have been made in the destination countries, for assisting immigrants and refugees. In this context, Lynne Healy highlighted the need for international social work in developing the links between domestic and global issues, supporting the argument that 'there is no such thing as purely domestic/local social work in 21st century' (Healy, 2004).

It is in the same global dynamic that one needs to consider the transformations in the economy of domestic care. It has been argued that migration responds to the needs in the West and leaves a care void in the East, where older people are less likely to find informal carers (Hochschild, 2000; Piperno, 2006, 2007). Migration simultaneously transforms the Western and Eastern welfare systems, which face an increased pressure for assisting children and older people (Andall, 2000; Ambrosini, 2005; Colombo & Sciortino, 2005; Zanfrini, 2005, cited in Piperno, 2007). The main message for social work is the need for integrated transnational policies that link the two welfare systems, the so-called 'transnational welfare'. At the level of case management, this would allow putting in contact the social work systems from sending and destination countries, for an improved assistance of transnational families. At a policy level, several authors (Piperno, 2007; Gheaus, forthcoming) argue for a system of 'Co-welfare' which consists in a 'shared responsibility' among Romania and the European states that benefit from care drain.

For the time being, in the absence of longitudinal research, the long-term implications for grandparents as primary carers can only be assumed. Future studies need to explore the changes intervening in the dynamic of 'skip-generation' families, with potential stable attachment bonds between children and grandparents and the sometimes-diffused moral sanctions applied to parents by children. In the Romanian context, grandparents' expectations of care at old age may be an issue. To what extent will the migrant parents or their children reciprocate grandparents' care, either personally or by transferring it to (paid) caregivers or institutions?

In many European countries, grandparents supplement parents in childcare or step in when more consistent needs appear (e.g. in the context of divorce or for children with disabilities). Existing evidence shows that on average, in 10 countries of research (Romania excepted), 58% of grandmothers and 49% of grandfathers provide some kind of care for a grandchild of less than 15 years during a reference year, with Greece, Italy and Spain having the highest rate of grandparents providing *regular* care (Hank & Buber, 2009).

The grandparents this research was interested in were facing rather unpredictable roles. They worked out their own way of understanding the structural conditions of the present and developed coping strategies. They comprehended and adjusted to the changes, being reconciled with the need for migration. The new ways of 'doing family' (Coontz, 1997, cited in Coles, 2001) are not without their shortcomings, however. They increase the vulnerability of elderly people who most of the times remain invisible when competing for social services along with other social categories, notably children they care for. Besides, the traditional expectation for the reciprocation of care remains problematic.

Acknowledgements

The author would like to thank editors Susan Lawrence and Sandra Torres and two anonymous reviewers for their helpful comments that greatly improved the manuscript. Special thanks are also due to Daniel Brett, Rosa Drown and Donald Davis for carefully proofreading the manuscript.

Notes

[1]   This affirmation refers to the temporary and seasonal migrants and does not include situations of highly qualified persons who emigrate permanently together with their families. The concept of *migration* inside EU is questionable, and officially to be replaced with *intra-European mobility*. However, this research will use the concept of migration in its non-technical and rather broader meaning of *mobility*.

[2]   European Parliament resolution of 12 March 2009 on migrant children left behind in the country of origin.

[3]   In approximately 25% of the cases when the mother only is migrating, children remain in the care of grandparents. This situation has been documented in other countries, as well (e.g. a double percentage reported for South America by Parrenas, 2001, 2005).

[4]   There are 3500 children in this last situation, accounting for 3% of all children with both parents abroad (UNICEF & AAS, 2008).

[5]   The average salary of €332.924 in 2009 (National Institute of Statistics) is associated with purchasing prices at European standards.

[6] The same scholarship argues that children do not always subscribe to parents' notion of better childhood, and depending on age, develop strategies to counter their actions (Dreby, 2005; Boehm, 2008; Horton, 2008; Lutz, 2008).

[7] Hochschild's position, although influential, has been challenged as being rather dichotomous (Lutz, 2008). The binary of 'care surplus' and 'care drain' was required to add the complexities of negotiation.

[8] This research is particularly interested in grandmothers, as they appear to undertake the care giving role most often. Nevertheless, the roles and the views of the grandfathers, largely underestimated in research and policy, require future consideration.

[9] In the paper, the reference in using the terminology is children. So 'grandparents' and 'parents' are in relation to children.

[10] The social characteristic of the grandmothers who were reluctant to disclose personal experiences may differ from those who did (in terms of autonomy as related to other family members, previous relations with authorities and community).

[11] There is, however, a process of accelerating ageing in the countryside, which makes a large part of the countryside severely isolated.

[12] In small towns or the cities, parents may migrate following the collapse of local industry. Multigenerational living arrangements are very rare. The changes following migration are limited to improved household amenities, payment of university fees for children and, at very best, purchase of a decent house.

[13] The names of caregivers have been changed.

[14] In Roma families, where the age at first birth is lower, grandparents are younger and occasionally migrate themselves for the common good of the extended family.

[15] Temporary migration. For the permanent migration, grandparents' expectations are different.

[16] This distance may be rather practical (children are living in the house of the other grandmother and expectations for mutual care are transferred there), or emotional (in the case of a mother who apparently would have been in the position to undertake the care, but chose not to).

References

AAS. (2008) *Propunere de LEGE FERENDA privind Ordinul nr. 219 din 15 iunie 2006 privind activitatile de identificare, interventie si monitorizare a copiilor care sunt lipsiti de Îngrijirea parintilor pe perioada in care acestia se afla la munca in strainatate*, National Authority for the Protection of Children's Rights, Bucharest.

Ambrosini, M. (2005) 'Dentro il welfare invisibile: aiutanti domiciliari immigrate e assistenza agli anziani', *Studi Emigrazione*, vol. 42, no. 159, pp. 561–595.

Andall, J. (2000) *Gender, Migration and Domestic Service. The Politics of Black Women in Italy*, Ashgate, Aldershot, England.

Autoritatea Nationalala pentru Protectia Drepturilor Copilului (ANPDC) (2007) *Official Monitoring*, Press release, June.

Boehm, D. (2008) '"For My Children": constructing family and navigating the state in the U.S.-Mexico transnation', *Anthropological Quarterly*, vol. 81, no. 4, pp. 777–802.

Cerami, A. (2006) *Social Policy in Central and Eastern Europe. The Emergence of a New European Welfare Regime*, LIT Verlag, Berlin.

Coles, R. L. (2001) 'Elderly narrative reflections on the contradictions in Turkish village family life after migration of adult children', *Journal of Aging Studies*, vol. 15, no. 4, pp. 383–406.

Colombo, A. & Sciortino, G. (2005) *Sistemi migratori e lavoro domestico in Lombardia*, IRES Lombardia, Milan.

Committee on the Rights of the Child (2008) Consideration of Reports Submitted by States Parties Under Article 44 of the Convention.

Coontz, S. (1997) *The Way We Really Are*, Basic Books, New York.

Dreby, J. (2005) 'Beneficiaries of Sacrifice: educational repercussions for Mexican children whose parents work in the US', paper presented at the *Annual meeting of the American Sociological Association*, Philadelphia, 12 Aug.

Gheaus, A. (forthcoming) 'Care drain: who should provide for the children left behind?', *Critical Review of International Social and Political Philosophy.*

Gomes, C. (2007) 'Intergenerational exchanges in Mexico. Types and intensity of support', *Current Sociology*, vol. 55, no. 4, pp. 545–560.

Hank, K. & Buber, I. (2009) 'Grandparents caring for their grandchildren: findings from the 2004 survey of health, ageing, and retirement in Europe', *Journal of Family Issues*, vol. 30, no. 1, pp. 53–73.

Healy, L. M. (2004) 'Strengthening the link: social work with immigrants and refugees and international social work', *Journal of Immigrant and Refugee Services*, vol. 2. no. 1/2, pp. 49–67.

Hendriks, P., Kloppenburg, R., Gevorgianienė, V., & Jakutienė, V. (2008) 'Cross-national social work case analysis: learning from international experience within an electronic environment', *European Journal of Social Work*, vol. 11, no. 4, pp. 383–396.

Hochschild, A. R. (2000) 'Global care chains and emotional surplus value', in *On the Edge: Living with Global Capitalism*, eds W. Hutton & A. Giddens, Jonathan Cape, London, pp. 130–146.

Hondagneu Sotelo, P. (1992) 'Overcoming patriarchal constraints – the reconstruction of gender relations among Mexican immigrant women and men', *Gender & Society*, vol. 6, pp. 393–415.

Horton, S. (2008) 'Consuming childhood: "Lost" and "Ideal" childhoods as a motivation for migration', *Anthropological Quarterly*, vol. 81, no. 4, pp. 925–943.

Joslin, D. (ed.) (2002) *Invisible Care Givers: Older Adults Raising Children in the Wake of HIV/AIDS*, Columbia University Press, New York.

Lareau, A. (2003) *Unequal Childhoods*, University of California Press, Berkeley.

Luca, A. M. (2007) 'Long-distance families', *Romania News Watch: Transitions Online*, [Online] Available at: http://www.romanianewswatch.com/2007/04/transitions-online-romania-long. html (Accessed 26 Nov. 2009).

Lutz, H. (ed.) (2008) *Migration and Domestic Work. A European Perspective on a Global Theme*, Ashgate, Hampshire.

Monk, A. (1990) *Handbook of Gerontological Social Services*. Columbia University Press, New York.

McGuire, S. & Martin, K. (2007) 'Fractured migrant families paradoxes of hope and devastation', *Family and Community Health*, vol. 30, no. 3, pp. 178–188.

Nesteruk, O. & Marks, L. D. (2009) 'Grandparents across the ocean: Eastern European immigrants' struggle to maintain intergenerational relationships', *Journal of Comparative Family Studies*, vol. 40, no. 1, pp. 77–97.

Parrenas, R. S. (2001) 'Mothering from a distance: emotions, gender, and intergenerational relations in filipino transnational families', *Feminist Studies*, vol. 27, no. 2, 261–291.

Parrenas, R. S. (2005) 'Long distance intimacy: class, gender and intergenerational relations between mothers and children in Filipino transnational families', *Global Networks*, vol. 5, no. 4, pp. 317–336.

Pham, B. N. & Hill, P. S. (2008) 'The role of temporary migration in rural household economic stratergy in a transitional period for the Economy of Vietnam', *Asian Population Studies*, vol. 4, no. 1, pp. 57–75.

Phizacklea, A. (1999) 'Gender and transnational labour migration', in *Ethnicity, Gender and Social Change*, eds R. Barot, H. Bradley & S. Fenton, Macmillan, London, pp. 29–44.

Piperno, F. (2006) 'Welfare for whom? The impact of care drain in Romania and Ukraine and the rise of a transnational welfare', *CeSPI*, [Online] Available at: www.cespi.it/PDF/piperno-welfare.pdf (accessed 26 Nov. 2009).

Piperno, F. (2007) 'The impact of female emigration on families and the welfare state in countries of origin. The case of Romania', *Studi Emigrazione/Migration Studies*, vol. 44, no. 168.

Ryan, L. (2004) 'Family matters: (e)migration, familial networks and Irish women in Britain', *The Sociological Review*, vol. 53, no. 3, 351–370.

Schatz, E. (2007) '"Taking care of my own blood": older women's relationships to their households in rural South Africa', *Scandinavian Journal of Public Health,* vol. 35, Suppl 69, pp. 147–154.

Silver, A. (2006) *Families Across Borders: The Effects of Migration on Family Members Remaining at Home*, University of North Carolina at Chapel Hill, Chapel Hill.

Soros Foundation Romania (2007) *Efectele migratiei: copiii ramasi acasa*, SFR, Bucharest.

Soros Foundation Romania (2008) *Effects of Migration: Children Left Home; Risks and Solutions*, SFR, Bucharest.

UNICEF & Asociaţia Alternative Sociale (2008) *Analiză la nivel naţional asupra fenomenului copiilor rămaşi acasă prin plecarea părinţilor la muncă in străinătate*, Alpha MDN, Buzau.

Westwood, A. & Phizacklea, S. (2001) *Trans-Nationalism and the Politics of Belonging*, Routledge, London.

Zanfrini, L. (2005) *La rivoluzione incompiuta. Il lavoro delle donne tra retorica della femminilitá e nuove disuguaglianze*, Edizioni Lavoro, Rome.

Žmegač, Č. J. (2007) 'Spanning national borders: split lives of croatian migrant families', *Migracijske i etničke teme*, vol. 23, nos. 1–2, pp. 33–49.

Families and caring amongst older people in South Asian communities in the UK: a pilot study

Christina R. Victor, Wendy Martin & Maria Zubair

The increasing number of older people within Britain's and, more generally, Europe's ethnic minority communities raises the need for the development of health and social care services which are appropriate to the specific needs and expectations of these older members of the various ethnic minority communities. Within the UK, the Pakistani and Bangladeshi communities can be identified as being in greater need of care and support in older age. There is, however, comparatively little research that examines the family and caring relationships of these ethnic minority older people, particularly those who are not identified from contacts with statutory and/or voluntary agencies. Drawing on a small but diverse sample of 20 older Bangladeshi and Pakistani women and men aged 50 years and older, we explore our participants' understandings and experiences of care and support within the context of their family lives and social networks. Our data from the 20 semi-structured pilot interviews suggest that, much like the trend within the general population, the family remains central in the provision of care and support for these ethnic minority older people. We conclude by considering the implications this has for social care policy and practice.

Background and context

It is no longer appropriate, if it ever was, to consider the older population of Great Britain, or indeed Europe more broadly, as ethnically, religiously and culturally homogeneous. Recognition of the diversity and heterogeneous nature of the experience of old age and later life is important for social workers both for the development of culturally and religiously appropriate services and their education and training/continued professional development. A key challenge for services—statutory, voluntary and private—is to develop a framework for the assessment of needs and delivery of services that reflects the increasing ethnic and cultural diversity of the older population of the UK and Europe resultant from the increase in both the absolute and relative number of elders from minority backgrounds (see Warnes *et al.,* 2004; Merrell *et al.,* 2006; Warnes & Williams, 2006; Gunaratnam, 2008; Worth *et al.,* 2009). This challenge is especially pertinent to the development of social work practice and community focused health care. Two policy drivers are especially relevant: (1) the focus upon delivering care as 'near' to service users as possible, rather than in institutional settings, and (2) the focus upon service users as active participants in the care process which means that social workers and other health and social care professionals are engaged in dealing with not only clients but also their family and social networks. Thus, it is essential to understand and contextualise the frameworks within which care and support are provided to older people from minority communities, how they live their daily lives and how this affects younger generations living within the UK and Europe in terms of expectations around the provision of care.

Understanding the family, care and support networks of older people from Bangladeshi and Pakistani origins is a research priority of significance when considering 'the futures of old age' within the UK (Vincent *et al.,* 2006) and Europe more broadly. Within the UK, Pakistani and Bangladeshi communities are notable for the very high levels of inequalities experienced (Qureshi, 1998; Harding & Balarajan, 2001; Nazroo *et al.,* 2004; Nazroo, 2006) both in comparison with other minority populations and the wider population more generally. These two populations experience considerable disadvantage across a range of parameters, most notably financial/material resources (Katbamna *et al.,* 2002; Phillipson *et al.,* 2003; Nazroo, 2006), high levels of emotional stress, especially for women (Williams *et al.,* 1997; Choudhry, 2001; Phillipson *et al.,* 2003; Anand & Cochrane, 2005; Lawrence *et al.,* 2008) as well as notably high morbidity rates for chronic heart disease, respiratory disorders, cancer and limiting long-term illnesses and disability (Katbamna *et al.,* 2002). These health problems are predominantly chronic long-term conditions that compromise the ability of individuals to live independently in the community by inhibiting the management of activities of daily living. In turn this may generate a need for care and support, which may be provided either by formal statutory services or informal family-based care networks or indeed some combination of these sources. Access to, and provision of, formal health and social care services may also be problematic because of difficulties in accessing information, lack of familiarity with available services, cultural stereotypes that influence the attitudes and behaviours of health and social care professionals and language difficulties (Norman, 1985; Katbamna *et al.,* 1998; Jewson *et al.,* 2003; Phul *et al.,* 2003; Owens & Randhawa, 2004; Anand & Cochrane, 2005). Research has predominately focused on the support needs and experiences of informal carers (Katbamna *et al.,* 2002, 2004; Adamson &

Donovan, 2005; Merrell *et al.*, 2005, 2006) and/or the relationships between informal and formal care services (Katbamna *et al.*, 1998, 2001, 2002, 2004; Sin, 2006).

Research examining the family and caring relationships of South Asian elders who are neither identified from contacts with statutory and/or voluntary agencies, nor because they have specific 'caring' ties, remains limited (see Harriss & Shaw, 2006). 'Classic' studies of family and social relationships such as those reported by Anwar (1979) and Shaw (1988) were undertaken when the Pakistani communities in the UK were fairly recently established. The preoccupations illustrated by these research studies were with community building, employment and education; issues of older age and later life were conspicuous by their absence although the innovative work of both Qureshi (1998) and Ballard (1994) are the exception. In this article we report some findings from the pilot study undertaken as part of our *New Dynamics of Ageing Project: Families and Caring in South Asian Communities*. We focus upon illustrating the range of understandings and experiences of care and support described by older people from Pakistani and Bangladeshi origins within the context of family and social networks, as this is a topic of particular relevance to the social work profession.

Methods

In this article, we report data from the first 20 interviews that acted as our pilot study. A semi-structured interview guide was developed on the basis of our key research questions and the existing literature (see Box 1). The guide was used to explore our participants: (1) social identities and levels of participation in transnational and local communities; (2) perceptions and experiences of family lives, social networks, 'place' and locality; and (3) own ideas, meanings and experiences of 'care' and 'support'.

Interviews were undertaken in the preferred language of the participant, and our intention was to record interviews (with the permission of the participant), with field notes being kept to supplement the recording. The field notes were intended to document details of methodology (how the individual had been identified for the study), details of the interviews (e.g. any interruptions or other relevant contextual details such as the interview location) as well as details of the substantive content of the interview. These were written up as soon as possible after the completion of the interview. Of the 20 pilot interviews, 1 was undertaken in English, 19 were undertaken in the participant's home and they ranged in length from 40 minutes to 1 hour and 35 minutes, with an average of around an hour. A feature of the pilot phase of our study was the significant number of participants declining to have the interviews recorded. Indeed, only two participants in this phase of the study agreed to the recording. Thus, our researchers took extensive notes during the interview and then wrote them up post-interview. In some cases interview notes were written down in Urdu/Syleti and subsequently translated—in others notes were written in English. This variability reflected the diverse nature of the interview experience and setting and the highly diverse nature of our sample of participants. The field note

Box 1 Interview guide

Biographical:
- What have been the most significant events in your life so far?
- Can you tell me a little about your life? For example, which places have you lived at so far, a bit about your family and about your jobs?
- Can you tell me who are the most important people to you in your life at present?

Migration history:
- What were your reasons for coming over to the UK?
- Did you face any difficulties here in the beginning?
- Have you returned to Pakistan/Bangladesh?

General overview:
- What sort of things do you enjoy these days?
- What is important to you in life at present?
- Is there anything in your life at present that worries you?

Everyday life:
- Can you tell me about a day in your life—what you do in your whole day, from morning until night? For example, what did you do for the whole day yesterday?

Family life:
- Who is in your family and where do they live?
- Who do you provide care/support to within your family? Who in your family provides care and support for you? How frequently do you meet up with family members?

Social networks and locality:
- Who are your friends/acquaintances? Do you know many people in the local area?
- How/where do you meet up with your friends, neighbours and acquaintances?
- What places do you visit in the local community? Do you like living here?
- Who do you provide care/support to among your friends and acquaintances? Who, among your friends and acquaintances, provides care and help or support for you?

Care and support and health:
- What does care and help or support mean to you? What sort of expectations do you have from your family/friends/people from the community?
- Do you feel yourself to be healthy these days? Have you had any illnesses? Who did you speak to about your treatment/condition?

Age and ageing:
- How does it feel to be ... years of age? Is age something you ever think about?

Social ties, sense of belongingness and well-being:
- How is life here in the UK for you, compared to what it could have been in Bangladesh/Pakistan? Where do you feel more happy and satisfied?

data were systematised into three elements: (1) standard demographic profile of the participants; (2) a discursive interview memo that summarised the methodological and contextual elements of the interview; and (3) the content of the interview either verbatim (from the recorded interviews) or in as much detail as possible for those based upon notes. The reliance on field notes for this article inevitably introduces limitations to the depth of our data and analysis. Interview notes lack the level of detail and richness of recorded interviews and are mediated through the researcher and their recollection and interpretation of the participant's responses. We were working with an under-researched group with little familiarity with the protocols and procedures of academic research (see Zubair *et al.*, 2010). The only means by which we could carry out our research project was to build up trust and rapport with our participants (and the wider community) during this pilot study. We respected their wishes for interviews not to be recorded and, in the main study, we were able to record the vast majority of interviews, as the communities became more familiar with our researchers and our activities. We acknowledge the limitation of field notes, which means that in this article we are presenting data that are predominantly the paraphrasing by our researchers of the participants' replies and are not verbatim responses. However, we believe that the originality and importance of our data make this limitation acceptable, especially as the content of the two recorded interviews echo the themes and narratives emerging from the other 18 interviews.

We wished to profile older people from Pakistani and Bangladeshi backgrounds living in the community but who were not, necessarily, service users or identified because they had specific 'caring' responsibilities. Participants were identified via the social networks of our bilingual South Asian researchers, links with local community organisations and facilities such as shops and snowballing. No participants were identified via the use of statutory services, either health or social care, although this did not preclude service users from participating in the study. Thus, a variety of routes and strategies were used to recruit a broad range of individuals to ensure that our study encompasses the diversity characteristic of these communities (see Zubair et al., 2010 for more details of our approach towards the recruitment of participants).

The importance of place and space in framing the experience of ageing is increasingly acknowledged as the sub-speciality of environmental gerontology demonstrates (see Peace et al., 2005; Evans, 2009; Smith, 2009). The location for our study was a medium-sized town in the south of England. Our study, unlike much previous research on ethnic minority populations, was not based in a metropolitan area such as London (Carey & Shukur, 1985; Qureshi, 1998; Gardener, 2006), Birmingham (Burholt, 2004) or Glasgow/Edinburgh (Bowes & Dar, 2000). This was because we wished to explore the experience of ageing for minority elders in settings where communities are smaller, more geographically dispersed and are less 'visible', and consider how these factors may enhance (or inhibit) the experience of ageing amongst minorities. Without the 'critical mass' evident in large conurbations, there might be less awareness of ageing issues amongst both the communities concerned and statutory services and, potentially, greater reliance upon family and informal sources. However, this focus had a number of methodological and ethical implications. The relatively small size of the communities made achievement of our sample size challenging; the dispersal of participants complicated the logistics of the study and the unfamiliarity of the populations with research meant that the fieldwork took longer to complete, as our research team had to develop a trust and rapport with the local communities.

We utilised Atlas.ti to systematically code and analyse our data. Our coding process involved various stages as we moved from very broad codes linked with key topics of interest in the study such as 'care and support', 'family' and 'social networks' to more specific codes, adding further new emergent codes as appropriate. Thus, the broad code of 'care and support' was refined into more specific codes dealing with the giving/receiving of care, expectations of care and support, etc. This allowed for the development of new codes and the identification of important themes relating to care and support and family and social networks, which are the explicit focus of this article. However, before we discuss the key aspects of our participants' under-standings of, and experiences of, care and support, it is necessary to establish the parameters of our study. These findings are preliminary in that they are based upon our pilot interviews and focus upon one dimension of our research project, the experiences of care and support. It is our objective in this article to highlight key aspects of this broad theme which we will address in more depth in future publications, in particular considering how spatial, temporal and socio-demographic factors contextualise and frame the experience of care and support amongst older people from South Asian communities.

Ethical approval was given for the study by the sponsoring university. All participants gave informed written consent to participate in the study. Our participant information document gave assurances of confidentiality and details of whom they should contact in the event that they wanted further information. Separate consent was sought to the recording of interviews. All transcripts/field notes were edited to remove key identifying information to ensure the confidenti-ality and anonymity of participants. In the main study all participants have been given pseudo names. Here we refer to participants in terms of broad age group and gender.

The characteristics of participants

Our sample of 20 participants comprised 10 from each of our two communities, with equal numbers of women and men drawn from each of the two communities. All participants were married with an age range of 50–76 years (see Table 1 for more details), and their length of residence in the UK varied from 9 to 42 years. The gender balance in our sample allows for the voices of both women and men to be represented

Table 1 Age, gender and length of UK residence of the Bangladeshi and Pakistani interview participants

Characteristics	Bangladeshi ($N=10$)		Pakistani ($N=10$)	
	Male	Female	Male	Female
Age				
50–59	3	4	2	1
60–69	0	1	1	3
70 +	2	0	2	1
Mean age (years)	59	54	64	61
Mean length of residence in UK (years)	22	17	32	30

equally whilst the age range offers the opportunity for those of different generations to present their experiences. This is important since the experience of ageing for minority elders is heterogeneous with gender, age and generation (amongst other things) contextualising the experiences of our participants. Whilst we cannot explore these issues in this article they will form key themes within the analysis of our main study and serve to remind us of the diversity within the population we are considering and older people more generally.

Family networks of older people

In order to contextualise issues around the provision of care and support it is necessary to establish the broad pattern of family, kinship and community ties within which the receipt and provision of care is played out. Transnational families, which may be characterised by the dispersion of the family, either nuclear or extended, across international borders are neither new nor the exclusive preserve of migrants (see Bryceson & Vuorela, 2002). However, research on transnational families/kinship ties has predominantly focused upon those of 'economically productive' age or the care of dependent children. Issues of care and support of older relatives both 'at home' and in the country of migration were identified by Blakemore (1999) and Wilson (2002) as important topics for research (and with important policy and practice implications). However, comparatively little research has focused specifically upon this area of interest (see Baldock, 2000; Harriss & Shaw, 2006; Baldassar, 2007; Zechner, 2008; Lunt, 2009).

Torres (2006) draws our attention to the (over) simplification of many aspects of the life and experiences of minority elders. One illustration of this is the easy assumption that the international family links of minority elders will be focused upon their country of origin. However, our participants reported family ties that are complex and include those back to the area of origin, links with children/siblings in other countries of Europe and globally, as well as extensive locally focused family networks and also family links to other parts of the UK (see Box 2). The web of family relationships for our participants did not demonstrate the simplistic model of a dense locally based family/kinship network linked into a network of family relationships in the area of origin as is commonly assumed to be the norm. Rather our data suggest a much more complex and dynamic web of geographically dispersed family networks, both locally and transnationally, resultant from a pattern of international and intra-national migration across the generations. Our participants had transnational family/kinship-based ties to their country of origin which could be weakened by the death of a parent whilst the migration decisions of parents, siblings and children have created, for this community, a web of relationships with a very broad range of countries. In particular migration decisions taken by children influence the continued evolution of these links, with participants reporting sons living in a range of European countries including Germany and Belgium.

Box 2 Key themes: social networks—field notes in italics

Family networks-links with South Asia	Family links-diminished links with South Asia	Family networks-links with North America	Family networks-links with Europe	Locally based family networks
Sometimes after a year and sometimes after two years [I go back to Pakistan]. *I like Pakistan very much. The life there is very good indeed* (Pakistani female aged 60+)	*I don't have much contact with Pakistan. Haven't been back for ten to fifteen years now because my parents are no longer alive. Before, I used to go to Pakistan every other year. Now we go to Canada more to visit my sister there* (Pakistani female aged 50+)	*We often visit my sister in Canada, and the one in America, and also the one in the UK* (Pakistani female aged 60+)	*My second son lives in Germany* (Bangladeshi female aged 60+) *My eldest son lives in Belgium* (Bangladeshi male aged 70+)	*Almost my whole* family—*almost all of it is here—lives in XXX. There are only two* sisters *in Pakistan. The rest are all here . . . (My) close relatives are here* (Pakistani female aged 50+) *. . . most of the* relatives *are here (in the UK)* (Pakistani male aged 60+)

Note: Words underlined were English words used by participants.

Experiences and understandings of care and support

Atkin and Rollings (1992, 1996) observed that informal or family-based care is fundamental to any community care policy for older people, and the contribution of the family generally in providing care is well established both qualitatively and quantitatively (Dahlber *et al.*, 2007; Pickard, 2008). Participants consistently nominated their family as the primary source for advice and support and the potential and actual provision of care (see Box 3). From a social work/social policy perspective, it is important to note that whilst our participants have strong links with their local community these may not translate into what is seen/ experienced as 'real' nor to actual care and support. The community provides vital resources in coping with living in a foreign land, provides opportunities for social engagement and offers support in times of stress such as bereavement or celebration such as weddings, births or visits from relatives. However, the community is often not seen as an adequate substitute for support by close family members, particularly the children and the spouse. Indeed this mirrors the situation for the general population of older people where the provision of a range of caring tasks—physical, emotional and instrumental—is largely the province of the family (see NHS Information Centre, 2010) and not the wider social network.

Box 3 Key themes: expectations and experiences of care and support—field notes in italics

Who provides support and care?	Expectations of filial piety	Inter-generational 'contracts' for care
I talk to the people who are closest to me whilst friends were just for 'time pass' (Pakistani male 60+) *Only your own people (meaning close family) do anything for you...only person that person will really help you who is your blood; any other person won't do* (Pakistani male aged 50+)	*If I need care I believe my children will look after me when I cannot do things on my own* (Bangladeshi female aged 70+) *I have helped them (children and their spouses) in all sorts of ways to settle in this country, so I am entitled to expect the same sort of assistance from them* (Bangladeshi female aged 50+) *I keep faith in Allah, that my sons will look after me and my daughters may look after me if their husbands are happy to do so. I like my sons-in-law as they do look after me too...I have finished my duty of looking after my children and now my children have a duty towards me* (Bangladeshi female aged 50+) *I hope my children will look after me when I am old and dependent* (Pakistani female aged 60+)	*I have four sons and one grandson. I think I am an old woman. I have the hope that my children will look after me when I am older. All my brothers live in the UK. Someone will look after me* (Bangladeshi female aged 50+)

Both men and women articulated a clear and unambiguous expectation that their children would, should the need arise, provide care for them in the future (see Box 3). Strong expectations of intergenerational piety were articulated and in some cases there were significant inter-generational ideas about 'duty' and entitlement for future 'care provision'. This may involve, for example, the transfer of material resources and/or the validity and recognition of previous and/or ongoing caring and support roles. At the same time family-based care remains a highly complex phenomenon that can be dissected and disaggregated into a range of components and which can be understood from a range of perspectives. For example, Parker (1992) distinguished between 'caring for' and 'caring about'. Zechner (2008) develops this typology further and distinguishes four distinct dimensions of caring: caring about, taking care, care giving and care receiving whilst Nolan *et al.* (2001) offer a model of family-based care that incorporates a temporal element illustrating how family-based care develops over time. We can identify elements of these differing typologies emerging in our pilot data, and we will examine these differing perspectives of care, understandings of care and the giving and receiving of care in our main study.

Gender is an important issue when considering family-based caring. In terms of giving care women were the primary carer for their spouse and an emergent theme, that we wish to explore in the main study was the reluctance to leave their spouse in the care of another woman, albeit one with a professional qualification such as a nurse (see Box 4). For widows or dependent women the primary source of care was often the daughter-in-law. Where married women were dependent, the daughter (or daughter-in-law) provided the intimate caring with the husband playing a secondary supporting and caring role with less intimate and bodily responsibilities and care, by contributing to everyday tasks such as food, shopping and dealing with finances. As with the example in Box 4, the role of the husband predominantly focuses on the external consequences of dependency rather than activities within the more intimate or domestic spheres. This seems to be in contrast to research within the UK where older men looking after their dependent wives predominantly engage in the whole range of caring activities (see NHS Information Centre, 2010). However, our older people were not simply recipients of care but they were also providers of care, mostly to grandchildren. Two distinct elements of this were evident—the active transmission of cultural and religious knowledge and practices and childcare-based activities, although they were often combined. Such childcare activities ranged from the irregular to the long-term and routine.

Receiving care from statutory services, particularly as a response to dependency rather than an overt acute/chronic health care problem, was both rare and seen very much as the last resort. There are clear issues around knowledge about accessing services and cultural appropriateness (see Atkin *et al.*, 1989; Gunaratnam, 2006; Worth *et al.*, 2009) and quality of services (Mead & Roland, 2009). However, our data also reveal the strength of the emphasis upon family care as the preferred option and the antipathy and negative views held about the need to access social care services (see Box 4). Having to turn to the State for care was clearly construed extremely negative by our participants, indicating lack of family loyalty and potential loss of face within the wider community if your family does not 'care' for you.

Concluding comments

Utilising interview data, mostly in the form of field notes, generated a number of issues that we will be addressing in our larger study. Thus, we need to interpret these initial findings cautiously as they are based upon a limited number of interviews. First the migration pattern of our participants meant that our study area was not the initial migration destination. They had moved around the UK before arriving in their current community, which resulted in more of their family members living throughout the UK. This was supplemented not only by links back to the area of origin but also much more globally; our participants had family and social networks that spanned the globe—with a focus upon the Indian sub-continent, North America and Europe. Thus, the family networks of our participants were highly dispersed with the resultant implications for both the provision and receipt of care. The family network is therefore not just within a locality which may have implications for access

Box 4 The provision/receipt of care—field notes in italics

Wives as carers	Daughters (in law) as carers	Using statutory services	Providing care
I provide a bit of care to my husband. He is ill—I take care of him (Pakistani female aged 70+) *I provided care for my husband for nearly 10 years. He died two years ago after a stroke. He could not move without help. I looked after him, lifting him, changing clothes, bathing him and helping him to the toilet. I enjoyed it because he was my husband. Allah said if you take care of our husband you earn God's reward* (Bangladeshi female aged 70+) *My wife is very supportive. Every time I go out somewhere, she cooperates with me a lot. Cooking and everything else, there is no problem at all for me. She helps me with everything* (Pakistani male aged 60+) *If I need any care and support of course I receive it from my wife* (Bangladeshi male aged 50+)	*I am totally dependent upon my daughter in law. She provides all the care that I need* (Pakistani female aged 60+) *My daughter in law accompanies me to the GP surgery and helps with buying medicine from the chemist shop and also sorting out the medicine I need to take each day. She helps me in dealing with the council. She supports me by listening about my worries and my illness.* (Bangladeshi female aged 50+) *My youngest daughter helps me in household work like cleaning, washing, laundry and cooking. She acts as my mother used to do. She massages my body on the days I really feel bad, puts warm patches on my joints and helps me in the bath and toilet. My husband also helps me by taking me to the hospital/GP appointments* (Bangladeshi female aged 50+)	*I hope my family will look after me otherwise I will go into a care home* (Pakistani male aged 50+) *When we have no choice—then we will use <u>social welfare</u>* (Pakistani male aged 50+) *My wife <u>helps me a lot</u>. She <u>takes me to</u> the hospital; brings me back. If I stay there, then she spends the whole day there with me—<u>looks after me</u>. She doesn't leave me dependent on the nurses* (Pakistani male aged 60+) *He did not want a nurse looking after him. He only wanted me to do everything, also I did not want another woman to look after my husband, so I did what made him happy. When he died we were all close to him. That is my peace* (Bangladeshi female aged 70+)	*From time to time I look after my grandson if my daughter in law has something to do in the after noon* *I have looked after my grandson who is now 14 since he was born as my daughter in law works. When he was ready for school it was me who dropped him to the school and picked him up and took him to the Arabic class. Even now in the school holiday time he very often comes to stay with us* (Bangladeshi female aged 50+)

to informal care, and social workers, especially those outside the major conurbations, need to be aware of the complexity and diffuse nature of these family links. Our pilot study did not reveal any examples of participants' participating in the provision of physical care to members of their extended family networks outside of the UK. However, there were numerous examples of the provision of material resources to help relatives, both young and old, in Pakistan/Bangladesh and concerns for the health and well-being of ageing parents. Both Baldassar (2007) and Zechner (2008) have developed typologies that attempt to explain observed patterns of transnational caring defined as capacity, obligation and negotiation by Baldassar and distance, resources and circumstances by Zechner (2008). We will be able to explore the utility of these typologies in our main study.

Second, all of our participants expressed an unambiguous expectation that their children would provide care for them in their old age. One Pakistani male nearing his 60th birthday contrasted the supportive but smaller community of mostly single men that existed 25–30 years ago with the larger contemporary community where *now they live just next door but they don't get the time to visit* (field notes in *italics*) and emphasised the importance of the immediate family by observing that now only the immediate family are likely to provide for you in old age. This is, perhaps, a surprising discourse that mirrors observations made by the wider general population where there is nostalgia for the more robust imagined caring community of times past. However, the expectation that the family will provide care is not unique to this community but mirrors the views of the wider population. Wanless (2006) reports that 56% of adults expect their family to provide care and support in old age. Finch and Mason (1993) and Finch (1989) have demonstrated the importance of family ties in the provision of care across and between generations (see also Ahmad, 1996; Adamson & Donovan, 2005; Ahmed & Jones, 2008). Not all participants were entirely sure that this expectation would become a reality (Butt & Moriarty, 2004) and in some instances care in old age was presented as in terms of inter-generational duty and entitlement. Our participants had been in the UK for an average of 25 years for the men and 20 years for the women. Male participants in particular commented unfavourably on the robustness and supportiveness of contemporary community networks with a previous 'golden age' despite the increased size of the population. Third, for those participants who needed care this was being provided mainly by women—either daughters (in law) or spouses. Unlike the situation for the general population, older men played little overt role in the care of dependent wives. We can also see the importance of gender relations in underpinning of caring relationships in the concerns of wives about having their spouses cared for by 'other women' such as nurses: a similar point was observed by Worth *et al.* (2009) in their study of palliative care. Social care-based services may be more appropriate and acceptable if they focus upon helping and supporting families to care rather than being viewed as substitutes or alternatives for family care. Friends were not seen as an appropriate source of direct care and, again, this is the case with the wider population. Whilst policy extols the caring capacity of communities, care for dependent older people is derived predominantly from the immediate family. Some concerns were expressed by our participants that things are changing within the South Asian community with one example cited of an acquaintance of one of our participants being put into an older people's home by his son. We will explore such 'generational tensions' in more detail in our future work.

Our preliminary findings mesh with those of Lawrence *et al.* (2008) and Worth *et al.* (2009) and support the suggestion that care giving is culturally normative: a position contested by Atkin and Rollings (1992) who argue that this is simply a way of limiting statutory support services. There were few respondents who received any form of formal care, apart from health services, and several expressions of reluctance to accept such services from our participants as these were implicitly seen as a failure of families to accept their responsibilities. However, it is important to contextualise such responses. Very few older people generally receive any community-based care services—at best 5% (Victor, 2010), and informal carers provide 90% of help provided with activities of daily living and self-care tasks. Whilst there are culturally based differences in the gendered provision of family-based care amongst our participants and overt expectations of care from the younger generations, the reliance of older minority community members upon their family for care and support has much in common with the general population. For all older people, regardless of ethnicity, the family is central to the achievement of the government's key policy objective of enabling them to live at home for as long as possible.

Acknowledgements

This study is funded by grant reference RES-352-25-0009A as part of the *New Dynamics of Ageing Programme* directed by Prof A. Walker. We wish to formally acknowledge the contribution of Dr Subrata Saha for her work on the project between October 2007 and February 2010 and who undertook the Bangladeshi interviews and six of the Pakistani interviews for the pilot study. Mrs S. Butt assisted with the translation of a number of these Pakistani interviews. We are grateful for the support and participation of our local communities and to all those who participated in the study.

References

Adamson, J. & Donovan, J. (2005) 'Normal disruption: South Asian and African/Caribbean relatives caring for an older family member in the UK', *Social Science and Medicine*, vol. 60, pp. 37–48.

Ahmad, W. (1996) 'Family obligations and social change among Asian communities', in *Race and Community Care*, eds W. Ahmad & K. Atkin, Open University Press, Buckingham, pp. 51–72.

Ahmed, N. & Jones, I. R. (2008) 'Habitus and bureaucratic routines, cultural and structural factors in the experience of informal care: a qualitative study of Bangladeshi women living in London', *Current Sociology*, vol. 56, pp. 57–78.

Anand, A. S. & Cochrane, R. (2005) 'The mental health status of South Asian women in Britain: a review of the UK literature', *Psychology and Developing Societies*, vol. 17, no. 2, pp. 195–214.

Anwar, M. (1979) *The Myth of Return: Pakistanis in Britain*, Heinemann, London.

Atkin, K., Cameron, E., Badger, F. & Evans, E. (1989) 'Asian elders knowledge and future use of community social and health services', *New Community*, vol. 15, no. 2, pp. 439–446.

Atkin, K. & Rollings, J. (1992) 'Informal care in Asian and Afro Caribbean communities: a literature review', *British Journal of Social Work*, vol. 22, no. 4, pp. 405–418.

Atkin, K. & Rollings, J. (1996) 'Looking after their own? Family care-giving among Asian and Afro-Caribbean communities', in *Race and Community Care*, eds W. Ahmad & K. Atkin, Open University Press, Buckingham, pp. 73–86.

Baldassar, L. (2007) 'Transnational families and aged care: the mobility of care and the migrancy of ageing', *Journal of Ethnic and Migration Studies*, vol. 33, no. 2, pp. 275–297.

Baldock, C. (2000) 'Migrants and their parents', *Journal of Family Issues*, vol. 21, no. 2, pp. 205–225.

Ballard, R. (ed.) (1994) *Desh Pradesh: The South Asian Presence in Britain*, Hurst, London.

Blakemore, K. (1999) 'International migration in later life: social care and policy implications', *Ageing & Society*, vol. 19, pp. 761–774.

Bryceson, D. & Vuorela, D. (2002) *The Transnational Family: New European Frontiers and Global Networks*, Berg, New York.

Burholt, V. (2004) 'Transnationalism, economic transfers and families' ties: intercontinental contacts of older Gujaratis, Punjabis and Sylhetis in Birmingham with families abroad', *Ethnic and Racial Studies*, vol. 27, no. 5, pp. 800–829.

Butt, J. & Moriatry, J. (2004) 'Social support and ethnicity in old age', in *Growing Older. Quality of Life in Old Age*, eds A. I. Walker & C. Hennessey, Open University Press, Maidenhead, pp. 167–187.

Bowes, A. & Dar, N. S. (2000) 'Researching social care for minority ethnic older people: implications of some Scottish research', *British Journal of Social Work*, vol. 30, pp. 305–321.

Carey, S. & Shukur, A. (1985) 'A profile of the Bangladeshi community in London', *New Community*, vol. 12, no. 3, pp. 405–417.

Choudhry, U. (2001) 'Uprooting and resettlement experiences of South Asian immigrant women', *Western Journal of Nursing Research*, vol. 23, no. 4, pp. 376–393.

Dahlber, L., Demack, S. & Bmbra, C. (2007) 'Age and gender of informal carers: a population based study in the UK', *Health and Social Care in the Community*, vol. 15, no. 5, pp. 439–445.

Evans, S. (2009) *Community and Ageing: Maintaining Quality of Life in Housing with Care Settings*, The Policy Press, Bristol.

Finch, J. (1989) *Family Obligations and Social Change*, Polity Press, Cambridge.

Finch, J. & Mason, J. (1993) *Negotiating Family Responsibilities*, Routledge, London.

Gardener, K. (2006) *Narrative, Age and Migration: Life History and the Life Course Amongst Bengali Elders in London*, Berg, Oxford.

Gunaratnam, Y. (2006) *Ethnicity, Older People and Palliative Care*, National Council for Palliative Care and Policy Research Institute on Ageing and Ethnicity, Leicester.

Gunaratnam, Y. (2008) *Improving the Quality of Palliative Care*, Briefing Paper, Race Equality Foundation, London.

Harding, S. & Balarajan, R. (2001) 'Longitudinal study of socio-economic differences in mortality among South Asian and West Indian migrants', *Ethnicity and Health*, vol. 6, no. 2, pp. 121–128.

Harriss, K. & Shaw, A. (2006) 'Family care and transnational kinship: British Pakistani experiences', in *Kinship Matters*, eds M. Richards & F. Ebtehaj, Hart, London, pp. 259–274.

Jewson, N., Jeffers, S. & Kalra, V. (2003) *Family Care, Respite Services and Asian Communities in Leicester*, 2nd edn, Ethnicity Research Centre, University of Leicester, Leicester.

Katbamna, S., Ahmad, W., Bhakta, R. & Baker, R. (2004) 'Do they look after their own? Informal support for South Asian Carers', *Health and Social Care in the Community*, vol. 12, no. 5, pp. 398–406.

Katbamna, S., Baker, R., Ahmad, W., Bhakta, R. & Parker, G. (2001) 'Development of guidelines to facilitate improved support of South Asian carers by primary health care teams', *Quality in Health Care*, vol. 10, pp. 166–172.

Katbamna, S., Baker, R. & Parker, G. (1998) *Guidelines for Primary Health Care Teams: South Asian Carers*, Project, University of Leicester, Leicester.

Katbamna, S., Bhakta, R., Ahmad, W., Baker, R. & Parker, G. (2002) 'Supporting South Asian carers and those they care for: the role of the primary health care team', *British Journal of General Practice*, vol. 52, pp. 300–305.

Lawrence, V., Murray, J., Samsi, K. & Banerjee, S. (2008) 'Attitudes and support needs of Black Caribbean, South Asian and White British carers of people with dementia in the UK', *British Journal of Psychiatry*, vol. 193, no. 3, pp. 240–246.

Lunt, N. (2009) 'Transnational families, older people and social policy: the case of New Zealand', *International Journal of Social Welfare*, vol. 18, pp. 243–251.

Mead, N. & Roland, M. (2009) 'Understanding why some ethnic minority patients evaluate medical care more negatively than white patients: a cross sectional analysis of a routine patient survey in English general practices', *BMJ*, vol. 339, p. b3450.

Merrell, J., Kinsella, F., Murphy, F., Philpin, S. & Ali, A. (2005) 'Support needs of carers of dependant adults from a Bangladeshi community', *Journal of Advanced Nursing*, vol. 51, no. 6, pp. 549–557.

Merrell, J., Kinsella, F., Murphy, F., Philpin, S. & Ali, A. (2006) 'Accessibility and equity of health and social care services: exploring the views and experiences of Bangladeshi carers in South Wales, UK', *Health and Social Care in the Community*, vol. 14, no. 3, pp. 197–205.

Nazroo, J. (2006) 'Ethnicity and old age', in *The Futures of Old Age*, eds J. Vincent, C. Phillipson & M. Downs, Sage, London, pp. 62–72.

Nazroo, J., Bajekal, M., Blane, D. & Grewal, I. (2004) 'Ethnic inequalities', in *Growing Older. Quality of Life in Old Age*, eds A. Walker & C. Hennessey, Open University Press, Maidenhead, pp. 35–59.

NHS Information Centre (2010) *Survey of Carers in Households in England 2009/10; Provisional Results*, [Online] Available at: http://www.ic.nhs.uk/webfiles/publications/Social%20Care/carersurvey0910/Survey_of_Carers_in_Households_2009_10_England_Provisional_Results_post_publication.pdf (accessed 18 Apr. 2011)

Nolan, M., Davies, S. & Grant, G. (2001) *Working with Older People and Their Families*, Open University Press, Buckingham.

Norman, A. (1985) *Triple Jeopardy: Growing Old in a Second Homeland*, Centre for Policy on Ageing, London.

Owens, A. & Randhawa, G. (2004) 'It's different from my culture; they're very different: providing community-based "culturally competent" palliative care for South Asian people in the UK', *Health and Social Care in the Community*, vol. 12, no. 5, pp. 414–421.

Parker, G. (1992) 'Counting care: numbers and types of carers', in *Carers: Research and Practice*, ed. J. Twigg, HMSO, London, pp. 6–29.

Peace, S., Holland, C. & Kellaher, L. (2005) *Environment and Identity in Later Life*, Open University Press, Maidenhead.

Phillipson, C., Ahmed, N. & Latimer, J. (2003) *Women in Transition. A Study of the Experiences of Bangladeshi Women Living in Tower Hamlets*, The Policy Press, Bristol.

Phul, A., Bath, P. & Jackson, M. (2003) 'The provision of information by health promotion units to people of Asian origin living in the UK', *Health Informatics Journal*, vol. 9, no. 1, pp. 39–56.

Pickard, L. (2008) *Informal Care for Older People Provided by their Adult Children: Projections of Supply and Demand to 2041 in England*, Report to the Strategy Unit (Cabinet Office) and the Department of Health, PSSRU Discussion Paper 2515, PSSRU, Canterbury.

Qureshi, T. (1998) *Living in Britain: Growing Old in Britain: A Study of Bangladeshi Elders in London*, Centre for Policy on Ageing, London.

Shaw, A. (1988) *A Pakistani Community in Britain*, Basil Blackwell, Oxford.

Sin, C. (2006) 'Expectations of support among White British and Asian-Indian older people in Britain: the interdependence of the formal and informal spheres', *Health and Social Care in the Community*, vol. 14, no. 3, pp. 215–224.

Smith, A. E. (2009) *Ageing in Urban Neighbourhoods: Place Attachment and Social Exclusion*, The Policy Press, Bristol.

Torres, S. (2006) 'Elderly immigrants in Sweden: otherness under construction', *Journal of Ethnic and Migration Studies*, vol. 32, no. 8, pp. 1341–1358.

Victor, C. R. (2010) *Ageing, Health and Care*, Policy Press, Bristol.

Vincent, J., Phillipson, C. & Downs, M. (eds) (2006) *The Futures of Old Age*, Sage, London.

Wanless, D. (2006) *Securing Good Care For Older People*, King's Fund, London, [Online] Available at: http://www.kingsfund.org.uk/publications/securing_good.html (accessed 18 Apr. 2011)

Warnes, A. M., Friedrich, K., Kellaher, L. & Torres, S. (2004) 'The diversity of older migrants in Europe', *Ageing & Society*, vol. 24, no. 3, pp. 307–326.

Warnes, A. M. & Williams, A. (2006) 'Older migrants in Europe: a new focus for migration studiesarticletitle', *Journal of Ethnic and Migration Studies*, vol. 32, no. 8, pp. 1257–1281.

Williams, R., Eley, S., Hunt, K. & Bhatt, S. (1997) 'Has psychological distress among British South Asians been underestimated? A comparison of three measures in the West of Scotland population', *Ethnicity and Health*, vol. 2, no. 1/2, pp. 21–29.

Wilson, G. (2002) 'Globalisation and older people: effects of markets and migration', *Ageing and Society*, vol. 22, no. 5, pp. 647–663.

Worth, A., Irshad, T., Bhopal, R., Brown, D., Lawton, J., Grant, E., Murray, S., Kendall, M., Adam, J., Gardee, R. & Sheikh, A. (2009) 'Vulnerability and access to care for South Asian Sikh and Muslim patients with life limiting illness in Scotland: prospective longitudinal qualitative study', *BMJ*, vol. 338, p. b183.

Zechner, M. (2008) 'Care of older persons in transnational settings', *Journal of Aging Studies*, vol. 22, no. 1, pp. 32–44.

Zubair, M., Martin, W. & Victor, C. (2010) 'Researching ethnicity: critical reflections on conducting qualitative research with people growing older in Pakistani Muslim communities in the UK', *Generations Review*, vol 20, no. 1, [Online] Available at: http://www.britishgerontology. org/DB/gr-editions-2/generations-review/researching-ethnicity-critical-reflections-on-cond. html (accessed 18 Apr. 2011).

Democratization of ageing: also a reality for elderly immigrants?

La démocratisation de la vieillesse: une réalité aussi pour les immigrés âgés?

Claudio Bolzman

Various papers published in Switzerland and elsewhere in Europe have highlighted an improvement in the living conditions of new cohorts reaching retirement age. This paper examines whether this general trend to old age democratization applies also to elderly immigrants. It reviews some dimensions of the older immigrant population situation in Switzerland. It explores mainly their socio-economic and health situation. The article also examines their access to social security and to social services for elderly people. It reports selected findings from two original surveys carried in Switzerland in the 1990s (Pre-Retired Immigrants study, PRI) and the 2000s (Minority Elderly Care study, MEC) on older Italian, Spanish and former Yugoslavians citizens who are residents in the country. The article gives also more general information about Swiss social security and social work with older populations.

Différents travaux publiés en Suisse et ailleurs en Europe ont mis en évidence une amélioration des conditions de vie de nouvelles cohortes qui arrivent à l'âge de la retraite. Cet article examine si cette tendance générale vers une démocratisation de la vieillesse s'applique aussi aux immigrés âgés. Il passe en revue un certain nombre de dimensions concernant la situation de la population âgée immigrée résidante en Suisse. Il s'intéresse principalement à la situation de cette population tant sur le plan socio-économique que sur celui de la santé. L'article analyse aussi les questions d'accès des immigrés âgés à la sécurité sociale et aux services sociaux pour les personnes âgées. Le matériel empirique qui sert de base à l'article est tiré de deux recherches menées en Suisse dans les années 1990 (étude Pré-retraités immigrés, PRI) et dans les années 2000 (étude Minority Elderly Care, MEC), sur des personnes âgées italiennes, espagnoles et ex-Yougoslaves qui résident dans ce pays. L'article fournit également des informations plus générales sur le système suisse de sécurité social et sur le travail social avec des populations âgées.

Introduction

This paper reviews some dimensions of the older immigrant population[1] situation in Switzerland. It explores mainly their socio-economic and health situation. The article also examines their access to social security and to social services for elderly people. It reports selected findings from two original surveys: the first on 442 older Italian and Spanish people living in Switzerland (Pre-Retired Immigrants, PRI research; Bolzman *et al.*, 1998)[2], the second on 290 older Italian, Spanish and former Yugoslavian citizens (Minority Elderly Care, MEC research; Bolzman *et al.*, 2003)[3] who are residents in the country. The article also gives more general information about social work with these older populations.

Various papers published in Switzerland and elsewhere in Europe have highlighted an improvement in the living conditions of new cohorts reaching retirement age. Many scholars consider this general trend as an indicator of old age democratization. Lalive d'Epinay *et al.*, for example, noted that 'the condition of the elderly population has changed profoundly. At the same age, older people now enjoy better health and are materially much better off. They report a feeling of well-being considerably greater than the generation of 1979' (2000, p. 377). The authors added that older people's family life had become richer, that they were more active and keen to take advantage of the opportunities available, and that they were more autonomous. In the words of the authors, there had been a 'general upturn' (2000, p. 378), but at the same time they recognized that sizeable needs still existed, particularly in providing support to the very old.

However, these findings concerning an improvement in the living conditions of older people were not, for reasons of cost and language difficulties, based on samples that were sufficiently large or representative of the population of former immigrant workers who reach retirement age and have to face up to the problems of ageing. These people, who mostly came from countries of southern and Eastern Europe, nevertheless make up a significant fraction of the working class in Switzerland, having been recruited for the most part between the 1950s and the early 1970s to do low-skilled jobs. The result is that studies on ageing in Switzerland largely fail to reflect the situation of a significant part of the older working-class population. This paper examines whether the general trend to old age democratization applies also to elderly immigrants.

Research into the relationship between age and migration has revealed a number of other factors suggesting that in studies on ageing greater attention should be paid to former immigrant workers and more generally to elderly immigrants. One such factor is that, contrary to popular belief, migration is not an interlude to be followed ultimately by a return to the country of origin. In fact, most migrants stay on after retirement in the society in which they have spent their adult life (Sayad, 1991; Dietzel-Papakyriakou, 1993; Tomé, 1998; Attias-Donfut, 2006; Bolzman *et al.*, 2006). As the sociologist Sayad points out, 'all immigration, even if purportedly for work reasons only (. . .), ends up as family immigration, i.e. basically as the immigration of population' (1991, p. 19). The other option is to come and go between the two countries, living alternately in the country of residence and the country of origin (Serra-Santana, 2000; Schaeffer, 2001; Bolzman *et al.*, 2006).

Research in Europe has also brought to light the more precarious living conditions of these elderly immigrants compared with elderly nationals. This situation manifests itself in different ways:

- A high rate of early exits from the labour market, for reasons of health (disabling injuries or illness) or long-term unemployment (Mehrländer *et al.*, 1996; Nelissen, 1997; Dorange, 1998).
- Financially precarious situation, the average income being lower than that of elderly nationals (Dietzel-Papakyriakou, 1993; Pitaud, 1999; Samaoli *et al.*, 2000; Allidra *et al.*, 2003; Patel, 2003); in this context, women are at a particular disadvantage (Torres, 2001; Attias-Donfut, 2006).
- Bad health, as a result of the harsh nature of the jobs performed (Scheib, 1995; Schmalz-Jacobsen, 1997; Toullier and Baudet, 1998). Bollini and Siem (1995) call this phenomenon the 'exhausted migrants effect', wherein these people were often selected by the host country just because they were considered suitable for the job.

In this paper we explore to what extent these findings can also be observed in Switzerland. Moreover, it is also important to examine which are the legal and real possibilities that the social system offers to older immigrant populations to counter precarious living conditions. Many scholars argue that a key factor is access to citizenship, that is, access to equal rights and recognition (Schnapper, 2000). However, according to Sayad (1986), as long as migration policies consider immigrants solely in terms of their status as workers, the legitimacy of the presence of elderly immigrants in the society of residence, and therefore the legitimacy of their rights, will be problematic. Thus, their risk of being in precarious conditions during their old age will be higher.

Demographic trends

Statistics on immigrant populations in Switzerland and in other Western European countries show that they are ageing or, to put in another way, that the proportion of those aged 60 and more is growing. Figures show this trend very explicitly. Thus in Switzerland in 1980 foreigners aged from 60 to 64 represented 5.8% of the whole resident population of this age; in the year 2009, their proportion increased to 13.7%. This growth is also clearly visible among foreigners aged 65 and higher. Their proportion among the resident population increased from 4.9% in 1980 to 10.8% in 2009 (OFS, 2010b). Examining more specifically Spanish and Italian citizens resident in Switzerland, they represented 3.2% of the 60–64 years population in 1980, but 8.1% in 2000, while among those aged 65 and more, these two nationalities increased from 2% in 1980 to 3.5% in 2000. The growth of the absolute number of Italians and Spanish older people (65 and higher) is more impressive; from 17,093 in 1980 to 53,098 in 2009 (OFS, 2010b). Their number has thus increased by more than three times in 29 years. The immigrant populations who followed during the 1970s and 1980s, namely the former Yugoslavians, Portuguese and Turks, are also beginning to show increased numbers in the older ages (see Table 1).

If the Italians and the Spanish represent the classical immigrants recruited as immigrant workers, former Yugoslavians and Turks represent more mixed groups of immigrant workers and refugees. In particular, the Yugoslavian group increased drastically during the last 20 years, mainly for reasons of family reunification and due to the high number of asylum seekers that requested protection during the war in Yugoslavia (Piguet, 2005).

If the ageing of immigrant populations appears still to be relatively modest, it is because on the one hand this process is part of a wider demographic trend, that is the ageing of the whole resident population. On the other hand, it is because immigration rates of young adults are still very important in Switzerland. Moreover, it is noteworthy to recall that available statistics take into account only older

Table 1 Foreign residents aged 55 and more, in number and in percentage of their national sub-group (1975–2009)

	1975		1985		1990		1995		2000		2009	
	N	%	N	%	N	%	N	%	N	%	N	%
Former Yugoslavia	579	2	2254	3	4828	3	10,766	4	8886	5	35,806	13
Portugal	157	3	788	3	1477	3	1932	1	2599	2	10,196	4
Turkey	314	1	1343	3	2307	4	3164	4	4251	5	7864	3
Italy	34,792	7	49,068	13	62,444	16	77,951	22	84,347	26	95,520	35
Spain	3354	3	8948	8	12,051	10	11,181	11	13,357	16	16,110	6
Other foreigners	40,250	13	49,464	17	55,298	18	67,577	19	85,804	15	108,259	19
Total	79,446		110,865		138,405		172,571		199,244		273,755	

Sources: Swiss Federal Office of Statistics (OFS), Registre central des étrangers, Bulletin d'information statistique, 2001 and 2010. Our calculation.

foreigners and not the whole population of older immigrants. The weight of the later is much more important, but those who became Swiss are not visible in the statistics.

If the ageing of immigrants is nowadays visible and starting to be acknowledged as a social reality, it is because a large part of this foreign resident population has settled permanently. One clear indicator is the fact that, among the 1,802,286 foreigners living in Switzerland in 2009, 62.5% have long-term residence permits. In the case of Italian and Spanish residents, 95% have this type of permit.

From invisibility to the 'discovery' of an elderly immigrant population in Switzerland

If the ageing of immigrants in Switzerland is the logical outcome of demographic trends and of their settlement in the country, as in most European countries older immigrants have until recently been invisible in health care and social policies. The hiatus between reality and recognition can be explained by different factors, among which the initial immigration policy and its effects have played a central role. In fact, immigrants who came from Italy, Spain or Yugoslavia to Switzerland during the 1950s and early 1970s were recruited as 'disposable' or temporary manpower, useful in the short term for the economy but not expected to be a permanent presence. They worked mostly in unskilled jobs and suffered severe legal restrictions. There were limitations on family reunification, geographical and professional mobility, and access to social security and public assistance. The immigrants also met hostility from sections of the native population. No integration policy was implemented at the federal level in favour of this 'first generation' of immigrants. This task was left to the immigrants' enterprise or to trade unions and nonprofit organisations (Bolzman *et al.*, 2004b).

When Swiss migration policy was brought up to date at the beginning of the 1990s, no mention was made of the question of older immigrants (in contrast to the reform of the German *Foreigners' Act* in 1990). For many years, the policy concerns in Switzerland with the ageing of the immigrant population have been mainly demographic and economic. In fact the presence of immigrants has been evaluated mainly in terms of costs and benefits to Swiss society, while the circumstances, needs and welfare situation of immigrant elders have not aroused much interest until recent years. Many Swiss politicians and social scientists view immigrants purely as a labour force that will help to rebalance the age structure of the population and finance the Old Age and Survivors Insurance Schemes (OASI). For example, in 1993 a member of parliament worriedly asked the Federal Council if foreigners needed to grow to 40% of the population in 2040 to finance the OASI. He felt that this would not be a solution, moreover, because 'these people ultimately grow old themselves' (Stalder, 1993, p. 40). It is noteworthy that the politician projected the phenomenon into the future.

At about the same period, the demographer Olivier Blanc (1991, p. 15) became interested in the socio-demographic challenges facing Switzerland including 'the aging of the resident population and the presence of foreigners that represents about one inhabitant in six. These realities raise delicate questions for society that cannot be ignored'. He went on to advocate a multicultural society. Blanc simultaneously considered the ageing of the resident population and the permanent presence of foreigners without discussing immigrant elders. By contrast, in a Swiss federal government report on *Ageing* published in 1995 of over 300 pages, there is not a word about elderly immigrants. In fact, immigrants were perceived mainly in terms of their economic roles as workers, consumers and contributors to tax and social insurance (Bolzman, 1999).

The designation of this category of the population as foreign elders or 'Gastrentner' (guest pensioners) sustains the idea that they are 'birds of passage' (Piore, 1979), not a settled population, a part of the national reality, nor necessary for social and health policies to elaborate special programmes to improve their quality of life.

The 'discovery' of older immigrants and their social welfare problems is thus very recent in Switzerland. Our PRI research on Italians and Spanish near retirement age (Bolzman *et al.*, 1998, 1999), carried out as part of the National Research Programme on Ageing, raised awareness of the phenomenon and led to an inaugural national conference on the issues in September 1999. That in turn was followed by different social measures and the creation of a National Forum on Age and Migration in November 2003. In neighbouring countries, such as France and Germany, awareness of migrant settlement and the presence of older immigrants arose from the discovery of acute 'social problems' among the most disadvantaged and the alert came not from research but from social and health workers in daily contact with this population (Samaoli, 1989; IZA, 1993).

Socio-economic and health situation of older immigrants

As in other European countries, the socio-economic and health situation of older immigrants is less comfortable than that of the Swiss older population. Even if the number of older immigrants is relatively small, they become overrepresented among the vulnerable, marginalised and precarious sections of the population.

Socioeconomic situation

Our PRI survey showed that some Italian and Spanish migrants had achieved better professional positions and that about one-third of the men and one-fifth of the women had become independent workers or assumed positions of responsibility by 45 years of age. However, when their situation on the approach of retirement was examined, it became obvious that some were in a precarious social and economic position or in outright poverty. A clear indicator is that a high proportion had been forced to retire early because of long-term unemployment or health problems. Men had been particularly affected; 20% of those aged 55–59 years had already left work, compared with about 10% of all of the residents of the same age (Bolzman *et al.*, 2004b).

In general, foreign workers have suffered more from unemployment than Swiss workers. During the economic recession of 1991–93, they were four to five times more likely to lose their jobs than Swiss workers (Haug, 1995). Today unemployment is still much higher among foreigners than among Swiss, although the overall Swiss figures for this are relatively low, 7.2% for foreigners compared with 3.1% for Swiss nationals in 2009 (ESPA, 2010). Long-term unemployment becomes particularly common between the ages 50–64. Only 36% of the long-term unemployed in this age group found a new job—more that 50% among the younger unemployed (Aeppli, 2006).

The main reason for early retirement is ill health. According to the MEC survey, a third of persons who had left the labour market before the official retirement age had health problems and 8% lasting unemployment problems. Two-thirds of the former Yugoslavians were forced to leave their work because of health problems, which happened to 29% of the Spanish and 21% of the Italians. In all groups, men are more affected by those problems than women (Bolzman *et al.*, 2004a). According to the PRI survey, the most severely affected foreign workers are those who had worked in construction, among whom one half received a disability allowance (Bolzman *et al.*, 2004b).

Immigrant workers (especially women and former Yugoslavians) approaching retirement are also overrepresented among low-income categories. The proportion of people whose personal monthly income is lower than SFr1000 and well below the poverty line was 8.4% in our PRI sample and 10% in our MEC sample[4] (about two-and-a-half times more than the resident population of the same age). A national study on poverty confirms these results. The likelihood of foreigners aged 60 + falling into poverty is twice as high as for Swiss nationals of the same age (Burri & Leu, 1997). This reflects the general situation of immigrants in Switzerland; the proportion of working poor within the foreign population is twice as high as within the Swiss population (−17.9% compared with 9% [OFS, 2008]). It is not surprising, therefore, that the foreign population appeals more frequently to the social services. In 2008, 6% of foreigners, as compared with 2% of the Swiss, received benefits from the social services (OFS, 2010a).

Health situation

Different indicators show that health problems are important among older immigrants. Here we examine two of them: self-assessed health and limits in daily activities.

Self-assessment of one's state of health is a subjective but reliable indicator of both physical and mental health and has become standard indicator in social research. A study from 1994 showed that 5–7% of people aged from 65 to 79 consider their health poor, and that is the case of 13–15% of people aged from 80 to 94 (Lalive d'Epinay *et al.*, 2000). The Italian and Spanish respondents in our PRI survey, although much younger (55–64), reported a higher prevalence (19%) of health problems. This score was very similar in our MEC survey (21% reported important health problems). But the situation of former Yugoslavians was even worse; more than a third among them reported bad health condition (see Table 2).

Another indicator examines limits in daily activities because of health problems. In our MEC survey we distinguished people that are not limited at all from those who experience a little or have a lot of limitations. The main difficulties in everyday activities are climbing several flights of stairs, moderate activities such as moving a table or pushing a vacuum cleaner and, to a lesser extent, shopping for groceries. Former Yugoslavians are really in a difficult situation with respect to daily activities. Almost 80% among them meet some limitations related to health problems, compared to a third of Italians and Spanish (Bolzman *et al.*, 2004a), and 15% of Swiss (Lalive d'Epinay *et al.*, 2000). This can be considered as quite dramatic because former Yugoslavians are younger than the members of the two other ethnic groups and the Swiss. We must remember that former Yugoslavians have the highest rate of registered disabled persons.

The problematic health situation of older immigrants has been described as the 'exhausted migrant effect' (Bollini & Siem, 1995). The majority of migrants arrived in Switzerland in good health, for it was mainly the more fit who left their countries of origin, and they underwent strict health controls at the Swiss border. After 30 to 40 years of hard work, difficult living conditions and insecure legal status, however, many are exhausted and have known health problems. A study in Geneva showed a relatively shorter life expectancy among semi-skilled or unskilled workers, that is, mainly immigrant workers (Guberan & Usel, 2000). Another survey of Spanish elders in Switzerland revealed that 30% of those surveyed were disabled or ill, and among those aged <65, the proportion was 44%. The majority of cases were related to industrial accidents or to the nature of their work (Embajada de España en Suiza y Femaes, 2001). In the case of former Yugoslavians, besides the problems of hard work conditions and insecure legal status, health problems are also associated with situations of war, persecution and violence experienced by refugees and asylum seekers in their home country.

Table 2 Studies on self-assessment of health by elders

Studies	Age group	Population	Poor health (%)
Switzerland, 1993	50–64	Swiss	4.2
Switzerland, 1993	50–64	Foreigners	7.6
Geneva, Wallis, 1994	65–79	All residents[a]	5.0–7.0
Geneva, Basle, 1993	55–64	Italians/Spanish[b]	19.0
Geneva, Basle, 2003	55–79	Italians/Spanish[c]	21.0
Geneva, Basle, 2003	55–70	Former Yugoslavians[c]	33.0

Sources: Vranjes *et al.* (1995); [a]Lalive d'Epinay *et al.* (2000); [b]Bolzman *et al.* (1998); [c]Bolzman *et al.* (2004a).

Welfare policy and the situation of older immigrants

Given the development and growth of the welfare state, social security has become the main means of protecting individuals from poverty and insecurity. Here we outline the Swiss legislation on social security, especially as it affects elderly people, and examine to what extent and under what conditions foreign elders are entitled to social security benefits.

The Swiss social security system has two aspects: social insurance and social welfare. The cornerstone of *social insurance* is the three-pillar system, organised around three methods of funding financial support. It is a threefold system of public, occupational and private insurance. Old Age and Survivors Insurance Schemes (OASI) and Invalidity Insurance jointly make up the first pillar, with pensions intended to cover basic living costs. When these are insufficient, there are supplementary benefits to raise income to the 'subsistence' or 'above poverty' level. The complementary second pillar comprises occupational benefit plans that provide old age, survivors and invalidity benefit payments (Bolzman *et al.*, 2004). The first two pillars together should amount to at least 60% of the beneficiary's most recent earnings and allow pensioners to maintain the standard of living to which they have become accustomed (Brumer-Patthey & Wirz, 2005)

The first pillar is compulsory for all, including the self-employed or people not in gainful employment (e.g. parents of either sex who take care of the home and children). The second pillar is obligatory only for salaried workers. The third pillar— individual provision to meet further needs—is optional but, unlike other forms of savings, offers certain tax benefits. The three-pillar system, embodied in the Swiss Constitution since 1972, is intended to ensure a decent standard of living for people of retirement age and other pensioners (Lalive d'Epinay *et al.*, 1987).

Social insurance therefore covers four main categories of social security benefits— for old age, for dependants (widowed spouses, children and the disabled), in case of sickness or accident, and unemployment insurance and family allowances. Since we are concerned with elderly people, we shall examine only the first two categories.

These forms of insurance grant financial benefits (pensions, compensation for loss of income) and cover costs in cases of sickness or accident. Social security benefits, in particular those granted in lieu of an income from paid employment, are mainly financed out of salary-based contributions. Health or sickness insurance, as it is called in Switzerland, is financed from individual premiums paid by the insured. The federal authorities and cantons participate to a greater or lesser extent in financing social security (old age insurance, invalidity insurance, sickness insurance). Supplementary benefits are financed completely out of federal and cantonal tax revenue. The occupational benefit plan (the so-called 'second pillar' of social security) is a fully funded system (Brumer-Patthey & Wirz, 2005)

Social welfare or social assistance is always means tested. Based on the principle of subsidiarity, it aims to provide everyone with the means to meet their basic needs, in particular people who are not covered by any other form of social security—those outside the welfare 'safety net'. To a large extent, social aid is administered by the cantons. Cantonal regulations differ widely and the disparity between the benefits granted is great. There are, of course, other cantonal and municipal institutions as well as private charities which supplement the two primary sources of social security (Fragnière & Girod, 2002).

Foreign elders in the welfare system

Today, foreign residents in Switzerland are net payers into the OASI scheme: they receive less than they contribute. However, the number of pensions to be paid to foreigners will rise sharply over the next few years because the immigrant workers who came to Switzerland in the 1960s and the 1970s will be entitled to draw their OASI pensions. However, foreigners' pensions are relatively low, since the amount of pension depends on the length of time that contributions have been paid, and most immigrants, even if they started to work very early in their lives, have worked for only part of their active life in Switzerland (OFAS, 2010).

The most significant difference between Swiss and foreign elders lies in their access to supplementary benefits. Since 1965, legislation has been in place for cantons and communes to pay supplementary benefits to those whose old age pensions are insufficient to cover their basic needs. These pension supplements are part of social security and beneficiaries are legally entitled to them. They make up the difference between expenditure and income. However, although they constitute a right, some may feel that this is a charitable dole and resent having to ask for it. In the case of foreigners, access to supplementary benefits depends upon nationality, length of residence in Switzerland and on the canton. Foreign elders need to have an unbroken 10-year residence in Switzerland to qualify for supplementary benefits. Those who come from countries without a bilateral social security convention with Switzerland must be recipients of an old age, survivors or invalidity pension in order to be legally entitled to them. Refugee elders, however, are entitled to receive these benefits after five years of residence in Switzerland (OFAS, 2010).

Unlike the OASI, the second pillar works on a money purchase system. Pensioners receive pensions based on the amount of money contributed by them and their employer into the pension fund, plus the interest yielded. Contributing to the 'second pillar' has been compulsory since 1985, but only for those with a yearly income of at least SFr20,520 (Art.7LPP). Thus, many women, especially foreign women, do not benefit from this provision, since they earn less than this amount working in unskilled and part-time jobs.

Health insurance gives everyone living in Switzerland access to adequate health care in the event of sickness, maternity or accident, where these are not covered by accident insurance. Every resident in Switzerland is legally obliged to take out this insurance regardless of age or nationality. Each family member is insured individually. The level of personal contributions varies from one canton to another and from one insurance fund to another, but the benefits of basic health insurance are the same. Within each insurance fund, the amount of contribution levied is the same for all members and no distinctions are made according to age, sex or nationality. Individuals may also take out supplementary health insurance which gives access to private or semi-private rooms in hospitals or to additional care (for instance, natural medicine). In the case of home nursing and care, the costs of assessment, advice and counselling, primary and therapeutic care, are covered by the health insurance fund. Foreigners are less likely to have supplementary health insurance than the Swiss, the main reason for which is probably its cost (Bolzman *et al.*, 2003).

In short, even if foreign elders started working at an earlier age than the Swiss, they would not fully benefit from OASI and 'second pillar' funding because they start to contribute to the Swiss system later in their lives or because they earn less than SFr20,520 per year. As has been noted, women are particularly affected. In addition, foreigners are not entitled to supplementary benefits if they do not fulfil the conditions of length of residence and thus they are more vulnerable to poverty.

Social services for elderly people and their use by immigrant elders

Since Switzerland is a highly decentralised, federal state with largely autonomous cantons and communes, there is no single model of social service provision that covers the whole country. Thus, most of the social services for elderly people are provided by local authorities. The only exception is elders' mediating services that are mainly provided by mainstream NGOs. Private providers are mainly involved in supplying specialised services such as house maintenance or equipment to assist daily living, but they also provide some other services (home care, day care, transport). Family members and minority ethnic organisations do not play any important role in providing social services or care; they act rather as a complementary support to other providers. As a matter of fact, ethnic minority providers do not play a major role in Switzerland in delivering services to elderly migrants. Most housing and/or care services are delivered by mainstream providers (Bolzman *et al.*, 2003).

The role of social services is to assist the socially disadvantaged in various ways, informing them about their social rights and about the kinds of services available to them, advising and supporting them when they are faced with problems, offering financial assistance, acting as mediators between users and institutions, etc. Public social services are organised normally on a district base. They are supposed to meet the demands of different kinds of populations living in a specific area. However, it is possible to find some specialised social services focused on the needs of specific populations, like women, elders, immigrants, etc. In the case of elderly people, a non-profit social organisation, Pro Senectute, is in charge of meeting their specific social needs and demands.

Pro Senectute has a central place in the national landscape of institutions that help and support elderly people. It has existed for almost a century. At the beginning, its role was mainly to give financial support to elders but, since the introduction of the OASI in 1947, the forms of social support it offered have become wider. Today, the main aims of Pro Senectute are to improve the quality of life of elderly people and to propose services that allow them to preserve their autonomy as long as possible. Pro Senectute tries also to promote an elderly persons policy adapted to our time and fights to reinforce solidarity between generations. According to Pro Senectute's annual report, 30,000 persons utilised its social service in 2005, 70% of them aged 70–89. The weight of foreigners has increased since 1999, passing from 8 to 12% (Pro Senectute Suisse, 2005, p. 5).

Pro Senectute offers lectures on preparation for retirement that allow elderly people to take into account the issues and modifications related to retirement in general, and to early retirement in particular. In some cantons, like Geneva, Pro Senectute collaborates with immigrant associations and social services to set up a specific preparation to retirement programs, adapted to immigrant communities. Until now, mainly Italian and Spanish elders benefited from these programs (PS Info, 2010).

Most elderly people, and older immigrants are not an exception, prefer to live in their own flats as long as possible, and social policies are oriented in that sense. The aim is to bring basic help and home care services to elderly people in order to allow them to continue their everyday life in their usual environment. Help and home care services are organised at the cantonal level. They are co-ordinated at the federal level by the Swiss Association for Help and Home Care services, founded in 1995. Within the cantons, help and home care services are usually organised at the district level. People of all ages are entitled to make use of housekeeping or household help and of therapeutic care. The services offer mainly bodily care and first aid, all nursing treatments, therapeutic care in accordance with medical prescription, support in everyday life activities, search of contacts with family and social environment, support during a convalescence period, and palliative care. Costs are paid for by the health insurance fund. Users pay a small part of it, which depends upon their annual cover plan. However, according to MEC survey, managers and professionals from Help and Home Care services estimate that immigrant elders are underrepresented among their users (Bolzman et al., 2004a). A study of the access of immigrant elders to supplementary help and home care in Basle shows that they know little about these services. A large majority think that the only possibility left to them is to spend their old age in a nursing home (Jacobs Schmid, 2001).

Day care centres are also oriented towards the support of elderly people living at home. They collaborate with help and home care services and with social services. Most of the users of these centres are women aged 80 or over. Day care centres are usually non-profit organisations that get financial support from the State. Thanks to this financial help, the centres are able to apply low prices. The price covers psychosocial follow-up and daily transportation for elderly people. It includes also breakfast, lunch and a light meal in the afternoon. Again, the MEC survey shows that immigrant elders underuse these centres (Bolzman et al., 2004a).

When elderly people become physically and/or mentally dependent, the main form of social support is nursing homes. These services are organised on a cantonal basis, but their way of functioning is relatively similar throughout Switzerland. They are provided with an important staff of specialised professionals (medical, social, housing, catering, administrative). Some of them depend on public sector, others on non-profit organisations, and some are private institutions. Nursing homes are quite expensive, since their cost includes medical and social care (medicines, apparatus, activities) and lodging resources (accommodation, meals, laundering). In general, the cost is financed by three sources: resident's contribution, health insurance participation and subsidies from the State. Many persons are not wealthy enough to finance the cost of their stay in nursing homes. In that case, they may ask for cantonal or federal supplementary benefits to the cantonal office for elderly people. Most of the residents are women. With respect to age, 78% of the residents are aged 80 or over. The average length of stay is about 38 months. The vacancy rate is very low, for instance 2% in Basle City and 4% in Geneva. Usually, waiting lists are long. There are no statistics on nursing homes' residents by nationality. Male immigrants are probably underrepresented in this type of facility. In fact, their life expectancy is shorter than the Swiss' one, because of hard work. On the other hand, according to some professionals, immigrants from 'South' countries would be more reluctant to enter nursing homes, since negative stereotypes have been developed about these places. Some cantons, like Zurich, have created recently 'Mediterranean nursing homes' adapted to the needs and demands of Italian and Spanish elders.

Concluding remarks

The socio-economic situation of foreign elders is strongly linked to the conditions in which they have lived and worked. They are overrepresented among the poor and the sick. They benefit from family and ethnic community support, but neither their children nor the members of their informal networks are able, in a systematic way, to take care of them in the event of disability, illness or other age-related problems. In fact, immigrants expect their main support in such cases to come from social security and mainstream services. Having contributed by their labour power to the prosperity of Switzerland, they believe that they deserve the support of health and social institutions.

Officially, most foreign elders have the same right to social security as Swiss elders. However, because of their shorter residence in Switzerland and lower wages, their OASI pensions and occupational benefits are lower than those of the Swiss. Moreover, they are not always entitled to supplementary benefits, even when their income is very low, because they have not resided for long enough in Switzerland. Sometimes they are entitled to benefits, but do not realise their right to claim them. Many elderly immigrants hesitate to ask for social welfare, even if this is a constitutional right offered to people in need, because they fear losing their residence permit if they need long-term assistance. In a way, elders who are foreign and poor are expected to find a private, individual solution to their poverty (Bolzman et al., 2004).

In Switzerland, a complex system of health and social care for the elderly has progressively been built up. Even if the mainstream providers meet most of the needs of the elders, their services are not always easily accessible to immigrant elders for many reasons: adequate information about services, adapted to people with other languages and with little formal education, is not available; no policy of integration has been developed in relation to this generation of immigrants; many immigrant communities distrust Swiss bureaucracy because of the country's harsh immigration policy; mainstream institutions do not pay enough attention to elderly immigrants; and there is lack of multicultural approaches in social work services.

In general, the foreign population hold a lower level of education than the Swiss, mainly because of the nature of the migrant work force recruitment. The PRI survey (Bolzman *et al.*, 1998) revealed that Italians and Spaniards aged 55–64 had a low level of formal education: 70% of them did not progress further than compulsory education. Most began working early in their life and many did not speak standard Italian or Spanish fluently, but rather a dialect (Bolzman *et al.*, 1999). The MEC survey showed the same trends for former Yugoslavians (Bolzman *et al.*, 2004a).

Immigrants have few dealings with public services. When they need some help, they turn to their family (especially children) or to trade unions. They seldom contact officialdom, either the social services or their consulate, and look only occasionally for advice or help from immigrant associations. Italians use more trade unions and 'patronati' systems for help than the Spanish or former Yugoslavians use their equivalents. This is probably because the Italian community in Switzerland is longer established and more structured than the Spanish or the former Yugoslavian ones.

In addition, contact with mainstream society appears more difficult in the Swiss-German region than in the French-speaking one, at least for migrants from Latin European countries. A survey of Spanish elders confirms this. Those who have most difficulties in speaking the local language live in the Swiss-German region: one third of them are not able to communicate in German and this proportion is even higher among those aged 70 and more (Embajada y FEMAES, 2001). Some hospitals use professional interpreters in order to ease the contacts between health professionals and patients, but such practices are less developed in social services. The problems elderly migrants have in accessing social services reflect the lack of any serious integration policy and illustrate the long term consequences. As stated by Hamburger: 'All the shortcomings of immigration policy are reflected in the social policy concerning elderly migrants: excluded from nationality, they do not qualify for the support normally provided' (1996, p. 41). In fact, many issues concerning elderly immigrants are deeply related to conceptions of citizenship. If immigration policies continue to consider migrations as accidents, as exceptions of a sedentary international order, older and younger immigrants will continue to be perceived as 'denizens'. That means that they will not be eligible for the benefits from full citizenship rights in their native or adopted countries: as a consequence there will continue to be 'surprising' discoveries of new generations of older immigrants living in precarious conditions. Hence, they will probably not fully benefit from the democratization of ageing. This hypothesis should be tested by doing more systematic comparative studies between national and immigrant elders.

Notes

[1] We use here the term 'elderly immigrants' in a critical way. In fact one can ask to what extent the term 'immigrant' can be applied to persons who are living in Switzerland for more than 30 or 40 years. But the term 'elderly foreigners' which describes the legal situation of these minorities is not more accurate to describe our population. However, we shall use both terms in this paper: the first when we describe sociological realities, the second when we refer to legal descriptions.

[2] The PRI research was part of a Swiss National Research Programme on 'Ageing'. It was a ground-breaking study in this field in Switzerland. Its aim was to better understand a phenomenon hitherto unexplored, namely, the ageing of the Spanish and Italian workers who had come to Switzerland in the 1950s and 1960s. A quantitative study on a representative sample of 442 Spanish and Italian workers aged 55–64 living in Geneva and Basel City in 1993 threw some light on these people's living conditions and their plans for the future.

[3] The MEC research aimed to know better the general situation of elderly immigrants in 10 European countries and their access to health and social care services (Patel, 2003). In Switzerland, three surveys were done between 2003 and 2004 in two regions: Geneva and Basle. The first survey was addressed to a sample of elderly Italians (100), Spanish (100) and former Yugoslavians (90); the second to 81 mainstream providers and the third to 25 professionals working in NGOs providing social services for immigrants.

[4] In the case of former Yugoslavians the proportion of people with income under the level of poverty was of 22%.

References

Aeppli, D. (2006) 'La situation des chômeurs en fin de droit en Suisse. Quatrième étude', *La vie économique*, vol. 10, pp. 30–33.

Allidra, N., Chaouite, A. & Abye, T. (2003) 'France', in *Minority Elderly Care In Europe: country Profiles*, ed. N. Patel, PRIAE, Leeds, pp. 33–51.

Attias-Donfut, C. (2006) *L'enracinement*, Armand Collin, Paris.

Blanc, O. (1991) 'Suisse 2000. Enjeux démographiques?', in *Suisse 2000. Enjeux démographiques*, eds O. Blanc & P. Gilliand, Réalités sociales, Lausanne, pp. 11–18.

Bollini, P. & Siem, H. (1995) 'No real progress towards equity: health of migrants and ethnic minorities on the eve of the year 2000', *Social Science and Medicine*, vol. 41, pp. 819–828.

Bolzman, C. (1999) 'Le parcours de deux générations d'immigrés: un chemin d'intégration?', in *Populations Immigrées: Quelle Insertion? Quel Travail social?*, eds C. Bolzman & J.-P. Tabin, Les Editions IES & Les Cahiers EESP, Genève et Lausanne, pp. 41–56.

Bolzman, C., Fibbi, R. & Vial, M. (1998) *Modes de vie et projets d'avenir des immigrés espagnols et italiens proches de la retraite*, Final report, National Research Program no. 32 (FNRS), Institut d'Etudes Sociales, Genève.

Bolzman, C., Fibbi, R. & Vial, M. (1999) 'Les Italiens et les Espagnols proches de la retraite en Suisse: situation et projets d'avenir', *Gérontologie et Société*, vol. 91, pp. 137–151.

Bolzman, C., Fibbi, R. & Vial, M. (2006) 'What to do after retirement? Elderly migrants and the question of return', *Journal of Ethnic and Migrations Studies*, vol. 32, no. 2, pp. 1359–1375.

Bolzman, C., Poncioni-Derigo, R. & Vial, M. (2003) 'Switzerland', in *Minority Elderly Care in Europe: Country Profiles*, ed. N. Patel, PRIAE, Leeds, pp. 193–217.

Bolzman, C., Poncioni-Derigo, R. & Vial, M. (2004a) *Minority elderly care in Switzerland*, Work Package 2, Final report to the 5th EC Framework Program, IES, Genève.

Bolzman, C., Poncioni-Derigo, R., Vial, M. & Fibbi, R. (2004b) 'Older labor migrants' wellbeing in Europe: the case of Switzerland', *Ageing and Society*, vol. 24, no. 3, pp. 411–430.

Brumer-Patthey, O. & Wirz, R. (2005) 'Comparaison entre l'AVS et la prévoyance professionnelle (PP) sous l'angle économique' *Aspects de la sécurité sociale*, no. 5, pp. 1–88.

Burri, S. & Leu, R. (1997) *Armut und Lebensbedingungen in Alter. Späte Freiheit?*, Schweizerische Gesellschaft für Gerontologie, Bern.

Dietzel-Papakyriakou, M. (1993) *Alter in der Migration. Die arbeitsmigranten vor der Dilemma: zurückkehren oder bleiben?*, Enke Verlag, Stuttgart.

Dorange, M. (1998) 'La sortie d'activité des travailleurs migrants', *Ecarts d'identité*, vol. 87, pp. 56–58.

Embajada de España en Suiza y Femaes (2001) *Análisis de la encuesta sobre la situación de las personas mayores españolas residentes en Suiza*, Spanish Embassy in Switzerland, Berna.

ESPA (2010) *Enquête sur la population active*, Office fédéral de la statistique, Neuchâtel.

Fragnière, J. P. & Girod, R. (eds) (2002) *Dictionnaire suisse de la politique sociale*, Réalités sociales, Lausanne.

Guberan, E. & Usel, M. (2000) *Mortalité prématurée et invalidité selon la profession et la classe sociale à Genève*, OCIRT, Genève.

Hamburger, F. (1996) 'Kommunale Sozialplanung für und mit älteren Migranten', *Zeitschrift für Migration und Soziale Arbeit*, nos. 3–4, pp. 36–41.

Haug, W. (1995) *La Suisse: terre d'immigration, société multiculturelle*, Office fédéral de la Statistique, Berne.

IZA (Informationdienst zur Auslanderarbeit) (1993) 'Special Issue', *Aeltere Migrantinnen und Migranten*, no. 3, pp. 1–130.

Jacobs Schmid, I. (2001) *Migration und Spitex Basel*, Fachhochschule für Soziale Arbeit, Basel.

Lalive d'Epinay, C., Bolzman, C. & Sultan, M. (1987) 'Retirement in Switzerland', in *Retirement in Industrialized Societies*, eds K. S. Markides & C. L. Cooper, Wiley & Sons, New York, pp. 103–129.

Lalive d'Epinay, C., Bickel, J. F., Maystre, C. & Vollenwyder, N. (2000) *Vieillesses au fil du temps. Une révolution tranquille*, Réalités sociales, Lausanne.

Mehrländer, U., Aeschberg, C. & Ueltzhöfer, J. (1996) *Situation der ausländischen Arbeitnehmer und ihrer Familieangehörigen in der Bundesrepublik Deutschland. Repräsentatifuntersuchung 1995*, Bundesministerium für Arbeit und Sozialordnung, Berlin, Bonn, Mannheim.

Nelissen, H. (1997) *Zonder Pionners geen volgers [Not pioneers, neither followers]*, NIZW, Utrecht.

OFAS (2010) *Statistiques de l'Assurance vieillisse et survivants (AVS)*, Office fédérale des assurances sociales, Berne.

OFS (2008) *Bas salaries et working poor en Suisse*, Office fédéral de la statistique, Neuchâtel.

OFS (2010a) *La statistique suisse de l'aide sociale 2008. Résultats nationaux*, Office fédéral de la statistique, Neuchâtel.

OFS (2010b) *La population étrangère résidante en Suisse*, Office fédéral de la statistique, Neuchâtel.

Patel, N. (ed.) (2003) *Minority Elderly Care in Europe: Country Profiles*, PRIAE, Leeds.

Piguet, E. (2005) *L'immigration en Suisse depuis 1948. Une analyse des flux migratoires*, Seismo, Zurich.

Piore, M. (1979) *Birds of Passage. Migration Labour in Industrial Societies*, Cambridge University Press, Cambridge.

Pitaud, P. (1999) 'L'accès des migrants âgés aux services. L'exemple du centre ville de Marseille: extrait d'une recherche-action', *Migrations santé*, vol. 99/100, pp. 77–96.

Pro Senectute Suisse (2005) *Rapport annuel*, Pro Senectute Suisse, Zurich.

PS Info (2010) *Quand la vieillesse est synonyme de problèmes*, no. 3, pp. 1–8.

Samaoli, O. (1989) "Immigrants d'hier, vieux d'aujourd'hui: la vieillesse des Maghrébins en France', *Gérontologie*, no. 70, pp. 32–37.

Samaoli, O., Linblad, P., Amstrup, K., Patel, N. & Mirza, N. R. (2000) *Vieillesse, démence et immigration*, L'Harmattan, Paris.

Sayad, A. (1986) 'La "vacance" comme pathologie de la condition immigrée: le cas de la retraite et de la pré-retraite', *Gérontologie*, no. 60, pp. 37–55.

Sayad, A. (1991) *Les paradoxes de l'immigration*, De Boeck, Bruxelles.

Schaeffer, F. (2001) 'Mythe du retour et réalité de l'entre-deux. La retraite en France, ou au Maroc', *Revue européenne des migrations internationales*, vol. 17, no. 1, pp. 165–176.

Scheib, H. (1995) 'Ältere Migrantinnen und die Altenhilfe. Untersuchungsergebnisse zur Nutzung von Diensten und Einrichtung der Altenhilfe in Frankfurt a. M', *Zeitschrift für Migration und Soziale Arbeit*, vol. 2, pp. 46–51.

Schmalz-Jacobsen, C. (1997) 'Veränderte Problemlagen und neue Projekte in der Ausländerseniorenarbeit', *BASGO*, vol. 1, pp. 4–6.

Schnapper, D. (2000) *Qu'est-ce que la citoyenneté?*, Gallimard, Paris.

Serra-Santana, E. (2000) 'L'éternel retour ou l'impossible retour', *Migrations société*, vol. 12, no. 68, pp. 77–84.

Stalder, J. (1993) 'Question ordinaire, 9.6.93: "40% d'étrangers en l'an 2040?"', *Sécurité sociale*, no. 5, p. 93.

Tomé, M. (1998) '"Os velhotes", les vieux Portugais de France', *Plein Droit*, vol. 39, pp. 24–26.

Torres, S. (2001) *Understanding 'successful aging': Cultural and Migratory Perspectives*, Department of Sociology, Uppsala University, Uppsala.

Toullier, A. & Baudet, V. (1998) 'Vivement la retraite? *Plein Droit*, vol. 39, pp. 50–53.

Vranjes, N., Bisig, B. & Gutzwiller, F. (1995) *Gesundheit der Ausländer in der Schweiz*, Institut für Sozial- und Präventiv Medezin der Universität Zürich, Zürich.

Social work, older people and migration: an overview of the situation in Sweden

Emilia Forssell & Sandra Torres

The globalisation of international migration is challenging social work practice in general and elder care in particular all across Europe. This article gives insight into social work practice with elderly people in Sweden by focusing on older migrants and their families. The article addresses the changes that Swedish elder care has undergone through the past few decades and how elder care is organised. The cases of two migrant families who care for their elderly relatives are described also in an attempt to draw attention to some of the specific challenges that social work practice with older migrants and their families can pose. The article argues that social work practice with these specific populations needs to become aware of the implications that understandings of ethnic 'Otherness' have for how elder care is planned and provided. Moreover, it is argued that the globalisation of international migration we are witnessing across Europe and the ethnic diversity in older populations that it brings about demand that social work is delivered in a more generationally aware way. Aiming to solely increase the social integration of older migrants can end up jeopardizing the social and economic integration of their families.

Introduction

This article aims to give insight into social work practice in Sweden and the manner in which migration challenges the context of elder care. The urgency of the topic is best demonstrated through demographics. Sweden has one of the oldest populations in the world. More than 17% of the total population is 65 years or older. Five percent is in the fourth age—i.e., 80 years or older (Larsson, 2007). A little less than 195,000 people of the 65+ years population are foreign-born (Socialstyrelsen, 2009). They make up 11% of the total elderly population in Sweden. The ethnic and cultural diversity of the 65+ years population in this country is, thus, far greater than some people realise. It is against this backdrop that this article will argue that Swedish social work is at a crossroads not only because gerontological social work needs to be developed but also because this type of social work must nowadays reckon with the ethnic and cultural diversity that characterises this country's ageing population (a similar case has been made elsewhere for the rest of Europe, see Torres, 2008).

Two specific questions are at the core of our argument: in what way do older migrants constitute a challenge to social work practice in Sweden and how can gerontological social work practice be developed to meet the needs that increased ethnic and cultural diversity in aging populations pose? In order to answer these questions this article is divided into four sections. First, the specific welfare context that characterises Sweden will be introduced in order to draw attention to the structural conditions surrounding social work practice in this country. The focus of this first section will be on the changes that have taken place over the past few decades; changes that are in different ways contributing to dismantling the Nordic welfare state. In the second section, the specific context that is elder care will be presented in order to give insight into the way in which social care for older people is organised in this country. In the third section, research on older migrants in Sweden will be presented. Some of the trends observed as far as the planning and provision of social care services that cater to their needs will also be presented in this section. In the fourth and last section, examples from our own research will be used to draw attention to some of the specific challenges that older people with migrant backgrounds pose to social work practice in general and to the specific context that is Swedish elder care. As the presentation of challenges henceforth will show, the globalisation of international migration is challenging social work to become not only migration-aware but also generation-sensitive. Hence, we will hereby argue that a deeper understanding of what the social position of ethnic 'Otherness' entails is needed if we are to formulate and deliver elder care services that meet the challenges that migration poses (Torres & Magnússon, 2010).

The Nordic welfare state: a backdrop for gerontological social work in Sweden

The Swedish welfare state has long been regarded as an archetype of the Nordic welfare model (Esping-Andersen, 1990, 1996). This is the case because of its high taxation and the fact that social security programmes reach large proportions of the population (Cochrane *et al.*, 2001). Since the beginning of the 1990s—and due to economic recessions—a rapid national deficit has led to cutbacks in all spheres of the welfare sector (Bergmark *et al.*, 2000; Palme *et al.*, 2003). It is against this backdrop that Blomberg *et al.* (2000) chose to title one of their articles about the effects that these cutbacks have had on the provision of elder care in our country: *The withdrawal of the welfare state*. International comparisons on elder care regimes and welfare state models still, however, give the impression that Nordic welfare states are different from other public care arrangements around Europe. In a discussion paper on the future of this model the Nordic Council of Ministers state that although 'there is more than unites than separates them in relation to the rest of the Western world. The Nordic welfare model is, however, more complex than the rest of the world readily sees' (Huset Mandag Morgen, 2007, p. 3). Thus, although the Nordic welfare model shares common values having to do with how solidarity between the generations and between citizens is conceived, there are, in fact, different versions of this model. These versions differ not only with respect to how they implement the value of solidarity but also with regard to how they translate the idea of public vs. private responsibilities into practice. To this end it seems appropriate to mention that the Nordic Council of Ministers has pointed out that other countries are in fact pursuing welfare policies that are more Nordic than those found in this part of the world.

Certain characteristics of the Swedish welfare state as it addresses old age are, however, still considered to be unique. The Swedish welfare state offers relatively comprehensive and high-quality public services to all citizens; its elder care system allocates services on the basis of people's needs rather than what their private finances determine; the system is characterised by both highly autonomous municipalities and extensive public home-help care services; adult children in this country have no legal obligation to provide care or financial support to their elderly parents (a state of affairs usually described as de-familiarisation) and the formal responsibility for the welfare of elderly people lies with public elder care and not the family or the individual. The fact that the system allocates services on the basis of needs as opposed to purchasing power is, however, one of the characteristics that have been questioned in the discussion paper compiled by the Nordic Council of Ministers in 2007. When summarizing the trends observed over the past two decades they write:

> The trend in recent years has increasingly been for private persons to pay for private companies to provide care. In the future we can envision models in which private persons pay local authorities/public providers and non-commercial enterprises for care services, either as a supplement to services financed and provided by the public sector, or as services that are purely privately funded for those who are entitled to publicly funded services. (ibid, p. 16)

Related to this is Szebehely and Trydegård's (2007) study, which showed that, in Sweden, although privately funded alternatives to elder care are still, if compared to Denmark, relatively uncommon, it is actually also clear that more Swedish older people—and especially those with higher education—utilise such alternatives. In other words, education and class play a role in the way in which older people in Sweden choose to meet their needs in old age (cf. Trydegård & Thorslund, 2010). Trydegård (2000), Blomberg *et al.* (2000), Brodin (2005) and Szebehely and Ullmanen (2008) have all shown that great inequalities exist due to class, gender, ethnicity and education. The seemingly comprehensiveness of elder care systems that operate under the set of core values underlying the Nordic welfare model has been questioned by Nordic welfare researchers over the past few years. The cutbacks have brought about what some refer to as the dismantling of the comprehensives that was characteristic of these welfare models. To this extent it has been shown, for example, that despite the fact that the number of people who are 80 + years old in Sweden has increased steadily since the 1960s, the elder care system has in fact become weaker and weaker over the past three decades. According to Larsson (2006), the number of people in special housing, the number of home-help care recipients and the number of beds in short-term care facilities within the health care system have all decreased over the past two decades. The period after the 1980s has, therefore, been characterised by increasing gaps between needs and resources. Both the actual number and the actual percentage of older people that receive elder care have significantly decreased over the past two decades. Over 60% of the 80 + years population received, for example, some form of elder care in 1980, while only 37% of people in this age group did so in 2004 (Szebehely & Trydegård, 2007).

Comparisons between the different Nordic versions of the welfare state suggest that Sweden is the country that has dismantled its elder care system the most (Szebehely, 2005). Nordic welfare researchers specializing in elder care are therefore beginning to question whether the role of the family in Sweden can still be described by the term de-familiarisation; a term often used to allude to the role that the state used to play in Swedish elder care. In this respect, the Nordic Council of Ministers states that 'relatives are increasingly subjected to pressure to assume greater responsibility. The scope of informal care is quite large. New systems relieve the state and the local authorities, but not necessarily relatives and those in need of care' (Huset Mandag Morgen, 2007, p. 39). Hence, when they describe the changes that have taken place in Sweden they acknowledge that the 'reduction in home-care services has increased the care provided by relatives and/. . . /to some extent this takes the place of public care' (ibid, p. 15). Some Nordic welfare state's researchers refer to Sweden's elder care system as an example of a system that is undergoing 'reverse substitution' or informalisation (Szebehely, 2003; Kröger, 2005). In this respect it seems appropriate to mention that the substitution thesis refers to the division of labour between family and state that has been characteristic of the Nordic model and the fact that in this part of the world there is an inverse relationship between service provision and family care. However, research on informal caregiving from a civil society perspective questions the idea that cutbacks in welfare state expenditure lead to an increase in informal caregiving practices and the taken-for-granted assumption that reverse substitution or informalisation can be equated with 'welfare state failure' (Jegermalm & Jeppsson Grassman, 2009a, b).

Irrespective of how increasing informal caregiving patterns are interpreted, it is still a fact that 'services have become more selective and resources have been concentrated to persons with the greatest needs' (Trydegård & Thorslund, 2010, p. 506). In this respect, it can be noted that a discourse analysis of Swedish policy on elder care from 1940 to 2000 has shown that the period that started in the 1980s was characterised by a shift in the way in which public and private responsibilities in relation to older people's needs were discussed (Brodin, 2005). Brodin argues therefore that:

...senior citizens' need for certain services, in particular those related to housework, are no longer regarded as a public responsibility, but rather a private manner that the elderly will have to solve, either by buying the services on the market, or by asking relatives for help and assistance. (ibid, pp. 204–205)

Our country's version of the Nordic welfare model is, therefore, no longer what it used to be. We have fallen behind all the other Nordic countries as far as the comprehensiveness of our system is concerned. This is why some Swedish welfare state researchers find it difficult to regard Sweden's elder care as an exemplary version of the Nordic welfare model these days. Hence, Szebehely (2000), Sand (2004) and Rauch (2007) have problematised the goals of our national action plan—which state that it is the older person's and not the family's situation that should be taken into account when assessing needs—on the basis of the fact that numerous studies clearly show that an increasing amount of the help and support that is given to older people in our country is being offered by the family as opposed to the state. With regard to the group in focus here (i.e., older people with migrant backgrounds and/or foreign-born older people as they are often referred to in the Swedish debate on elder care), this raises the question of what decreasing public support and increasing expectations on family dependency could end up meaning for migrant families.

Gerontological social work in Sweden: a general look at the context of elder care

Understanding how social work with older people in general and older migrants in particular is delivered in Sweden requires insight into the way in which the elder care system operates more generally. The first thing to be stated is that the responsibility for the welfare of elderly people in Sweden is divided between three levels of government. At the national level it is the parliament and the government that set out policies and directives by means of, for example, legislation. At the regional level, the county councils or regions (there are 21 of those) are responsible for the provision of health and medical care while at the local level, it is the municipalities (290 in all) that are legally obliged to meet the social care, nursing and housing needs of elderly people. The Ministry of Health and Social Affairs of the Government Offices of Sweden describes elder care by stating that the general guiding principles are that 'social care and health care for the elderly are primarily public sector tasks and that care is to be provided by trained and qualified staff' (Regeringskansliet, 2007, p. 1). They state also that 'one of the most important principles of Swedish policy for the elderly is that public action is to be framed in such way that older people can continue living in their own homes for as long as possible, even when in need of extensive health care and social care' (ibid). In light of the cutbacks alluded to in the previous section it seems appropriate to question whether these ambitious goals are, in fact, attainable.

An extensive set of rules and regulations governs and influences social work practice with older people in this country. The most important ones are the Social Services Act (SFS 2001: 453), the Health Care Act (SFS 1982: 763), the Municipality

Act (SFS 1991: 900) and the Act concerning Support and Service for Persons with Certain Functional Impairments (LSS 1993: 387). Two major laws guide the actual provision of care to older people in Sweden. These are the Health and Medical Services Act of 1983 (which states that care shall be available to all, irrespective of income, age or residence) and the Social Services Act of 1982 (which was revised in 2001 and grants people assistance with their livelihood as well as other aspects of living if their needs cannot be met through other means). Both of these laws are often described as framework laws, meaning that although they include some elements of detailed regulation, they do allow for local autonomy in decision-making. Something else worth mentioning is that these laws cannot guarantee that equality exists in the manner in which care is provided in our country. It is for this reason that Bergmark *et al.* (2000) have argued that although Sweden's welfare policy is characterised by the concept of universality, there has always been acceptance for needs assessment for many services. The Social Service Act's statement that states specifically that assistance is provided reads: 'if needs cannot be provided for in any other way' (own translation). This statement gives the municipalities much leeway for interpretation. There are, therefore, numerous differences between municipalities when it comes to coverage rates, eligibility criteria, the fees they take for the services they provide and even the quality of the care that they offer (ibid). A recent study shows, however, that although the 1990s were characterised by high degrees of decentralisation, we are now witnessing more streamlining and uniformity in the manner in which municipalities adjust to the national average (Trydegård & Thorslund, 2010).

Organisationally, social work services are delivered through two very specific administrative units. These go under the heading of 'individual and family care' (hereby alluded to as IFC and in Swedish called 'individ och familjomsorg') which focuses on children and adults up until the age of 65 years, and 'handicap and elder care' (HEC, which in Swedish is called 'hadikapp och äldreomsorg'). This division of labour presupposes an age-based understanding of the target groups with which social work is concerned; a division of labour that we will henceforth show to be problematic when addressing the needs of older migrants and their families. Access to social work services in Sweden is not, however, conditioned by citizenship, country of origin or length of residence. This means that older people with migrant backgrounds who have a resident permit can seek the services that are offered.

Having given some insight into how the Swedish system works it seems important to stress that social work with older people in this country continues to be about *social care* rather than *change,* which is what social work normally focuses on when the target group is younger. The most common social work practice with older people is therefore needs assessment. Needs assessors (or care managers as they are sometimes called) conduct an evaluation of abilities and an assessment of expressed needs. If deemed eligible the process leads to the approval of elder care services (i.e., safety alarm, short-term care or special housing for the elderly or home-help care). Elder care recipients are charged a fee for the services for which they have been approved. Fees are set according to the recipient's income—the smaller the income, the lower the fee. Sometimes, older people's relatives are employed as home-helpers. This means that they are formally employed by the elder care system even though in practice they are only serving the needs of their own older relatives. Another form of support is home care grants. These are paid directly to the person in need of care who uses it to pay their helpers. The authorities are not informed about who performs the care in such cases, or how the parties are affected.

Of interest to a special issue such as this one is perhaps that need assessors have different educational backgrounds. Most need assessors are trained in social work and/or in social care sciences. This means that they are not necessarily knowledgeable enough about some of the specific old-age related needs of the clients they are meant to serve. Some municipalities in Sweden have therefore started to recruit nurses and other health-related occupations to care management/need assessment positions (Andersson, 2007). The sentiment seems to be that as elder care has changed (and we have moved toward less home-help services being made available to elderly people with less acute needs), new qualifications are needed. In this situation, need assessors need to collaborate more closely with the health care system. Their role is therefore crucial and complex since these are the people that implement the relatively non-specific framework law that regulates elder care recipiency in this country (cf. Dunér, 2005). It is for this reason that numerous Swedish dissertations in social work have focused on the negotiations that take place between older people in need of help and support who seek elder care services and need assessors (cf. Blomberg, 2004; Lindelöf & Rönnbäck, 2004; Janlöv, 2006; Olaison, 2009). All of these dissertations argue that what need assessors assess is not older people's needs per se but rather what they are able to convey as a legitimate enough need. On the basis of an extensive communication study on assessment talk, Olaison (2009) has convincingly shown that in order to be perceived as an eligible elder care recipient in Sweden today, an older person cannot just be in need of help, they need also to be an eloquently gifted person who is successful in both, establishing him/herself as a potential client and expressing their needs in a convincing enough manner so that they can be deemed worthy of public care and support. This suggests that those who do not command the Swedish language and/or who are unfamiliar with the Swedish system run the risk of being disadvantaged in the need assessment process.

Due to the cutbacks alluded to earlier, the thresholds for both needs assessments and means testing have been raised. An individual must have greater needs and less means to qualify these days. Phrased differently, Sundström and Johansson (2005) have argued that because the Social Welfare Act is in fact very vague as far as stating the obligations that municipalities have, it 'has recently been interpreted, with dubious legality, to the effect that elders who have offspring or other family living nearby, or who are well-to-do, are denied public help (ibid, p. S8). This interpretation seems particularly problematic for older migrants and their families as the cases drawn from our own research in the last section of this article will show.

Social work with migrants: alternative elder care in the making

The Swedish welfare state is nowadays very much concerned with the increasing number of multi-diseased and functionally impaired people whose future needs for health and social care must be met. The increased ethnic and cultural diversity that characterises Swedish society today is also a source of concern. In 2009 the Swedish Government appointed a special commission whose task was to describe the challenges that social work practice faces when dealing with clients whose cultural background is not Swedish, who have insufficient knowledge of the Swedish language and/or who lack knowledge of Swedish society (Socialstyrelsen, 2010). Alarmingly enough, the written report that this commission produced only mentions older migrants once and does so by alluding not to their needs per se but to the challenges they pose to the integration of the younger migrant generation (e.g., Edström, 2008). Two other interesting things can be mentioned in regard to this report: first, the commission's description of social work relegates elder care services to the periphery of this practice, and second, migrants are assumed to be young. The report is, therefore, a testament to the old age *and* migration obliviousness that is characteristic of Swedish social work; a characteristic that is in fact inhibiting the sector from developing practices that can meet the needs of older migrants and their families. It is for this reason that the National Board of Health and Welfare has urged the practice of social work to increase its migration-awareness.

Despite this report's failure to address the specific needs of older migrants, it is clear that the growing ethnic and cultural diversity among elderly people in Sweden has led to an increase in different care options, such as special housing for older people who share the same ethnic background or language (Magnùsson, 2007; Heikkilä, 2010). However, older people born abroad still utilise public elder care to a lesser extent than their Swedish counterparts (Gunnarsson, 2002); 19.7% of older people born abroad receive public elder care, compared to 23% of those who are Swedish-born (USK, 2009, in Torres, 2010b). They are also under-represented in special residences and, as already stated, are strongly over-represented as recipients of home care grants (Forsell, 2004; Socialstyrelsen, 2009). This illustrates one of the challenges with which this article is concerned namely, that 'special' care arrangements are being created in Sweden in order to meet the needs that the increasing ethnic and cultural diversity of the population have and that these arrangements are often performed in an unregulated way since they are in fact relegated to the periphery of the welfare state.

To this end it must be mentioned that many migrant families have little knowledge of the welfare state's organisations, rules and regulations. This may be the reason why they often activate their informal networks when care needs arise. This situation is not, however, unique for this group of older people. As stated earlier, the vast majority of care provided to older people in Sweden—irrespective of ethnic background—is actually provided by informal caregivers, often next of kin (Johansson, 2007). What is unique in migrant families is not that they engage in informal care but that they may do so because they lack both the language and the knowledge necessary to find out that there are other elder care arrangements available. Research also suggests that past experiences of bad treatment in encounters with Swedish social workers or public care have made some migrant families sceptical of the system (Forssell, 2004, 2006; Heikkilä, 2004).

In this respect it must be mentioned that research has shown on numerous occasions that migrants are often regarded as ethnic 'Others' in this country (e.g., Mattsson, 2001; Bredström, 2002; Brune, 2008). As such they are believed to be fundamentally different from Swedes which is why they are often regarded as aberrations from the norm whose difference is deemed explainable first and foremost through their ethnic and cultural background. Migration researchers in Sweden describe therefore the way in which societal institutions regard migrants as prime examples of culturalist practice (Ålund & Schierup 1991; Johansson, 2010). Against this backdrop it is understandable that research has also shown that the institutional category often referred to as 'older migrants' in old age policy is a category under construction in Swedish elder care research, policy and practice (Ronström, 2002; Torres, 2006). Thus, older migrants are often regarded as a homogenous category whose most interesting source of difference is their non-Swedishness. As such, they are believed to have 'special needs' that challenge Swedish elder care. This means that their diversity is seldom acknowledged. Instead it is their difference that is often in focus. Hence Torres (2006) has suggested that older migrants are 'Othered' on the basis of their age by Swedish policy that focuses on migrants (as the report on the commission mentioned above clearly illustrates) as well as on the basis of their ethnic 'Otherness' by old-age policy. With regards to the latter, Machat (2010) has shown— after deconstructing the discourse utilised in Swedish social policy on old age—that policy documents make a distinction between 'our' elders (i.e., Swedes) and 'their' elders (i.e., migrants). We therefore suggest that the user/agency-oriented perspective in social work with elderly people that is widespread in Sweden at present (Socialstyrelsen, 2006) does not seem to include migrants. Therefore, older migrants run the risk of falling between the cracks of Swedish social work practice since they are neither typical for their age nor typical for their social position of ethnic 'Otherness' as that position is regarded in this country (i.e., as a position that is often assumed to come together with young age).

Older migrants and their families: a challenge to social work practice in Sweden

In this section, we will allude to two examples drawn from our own research (e.g., Forssell, 2004) which show that the innovative ways in which older migrants and their families handle increasing care needs can lead to arrangements that solve their own families' needs but pose new challenges to social work practice with the younger generation. The first example is about Maria, a middle-aged woman cohabiting with and caring for her aged husband and mother, both late-in-life migrants. Her mother has a home care grant and that is what pays for the care that Maria provides. Maria's husband is severely disabled and requires care as well. However, his care needs have not been assessed. When Maria is asked to talk about his situation she says: 'I am already at home helping mother, why should my husband apply for needs assessment?' Maria's mother and husband seldom leave the home. Maria left her low-paid full-time job in order to look after them, thereby losing her income. She has been granted maintenance support from social services as compensation. Every month a sum is deducted from the maintenance support she receives, which corresponds to the mother's home care grant.

Maria's pre-informal care situation—i.e., before she quit her job to care for her mother and husband—could be described as one of social and economic integration. Once her mother and husband's care needs increased and Maria felt that she had little option but to step in as an informal caregiver to both of them, her situation changed. Describing her present situation as one of social integration is not really possible at this point in time since her care burden relegates her to her home. Something else worth mentioning is that Maria sought help from social services for her mother who was in fact awarded a place in a home for elderly people. Language and cultural barriers led to a lack of social integration for Maria's mother in that home. On numerous occasions while her mother was living there Maria was called by the staff who could not communicate with her mother and who, as a result of this, did not feel they could provide the help that she needed. The fact that Maria's mother did not wish to be in the home complicated matters. Sweden's elder care rules state that it is older people themselves who should decide about their situation. Keeping Maria's mother in the home against her will was therefore not possible. Maria's will or needs were, therefore, not taken into consideration.

Related to this is the fact that research on elder care staff expectations of migrant families shows that it is not uncommon for social services to expect migrant families to step in as informal caregivers (cf. Forssell, 2010; Torres, 2010a). Hence, it comes as no surprise to hear that when Maria sought help from social services for her mother she was admonished for not stepping in. This family's case is an example of not only the lack of social and economic integration that migrant families risk when their caregiving burden increases but also an example of the vulnerable situation in which late-in-life migrants can find themselves when the system cannot provide the cultural and language-appropriate care that some of them need. When Maria and her mother's case are handled as separate entities, social work practice is also not only insufficiently meeting their needs but also worsening their situation since the mother's social integration leads to the daughter's lack of such. The fact that Maria meets the care needs of two elderly people, around the clock, at a cost to the municipality corresponding to the maintenance support for one person raises the question of whether the decisions made in her case are a testament to both crass economic logic and the culturalist regard that research has shown to be characteristic of Swedish social services.

The other example concerns a young girl, Fadwa, who lives with her paternal grandmother in a room with a kitchenette in special accommodation for elderly people with special needs. Fadwa's grandmother is functionally disabled and suffers from several illnesses requiring frequent and regular medication. She does not receive help from the staff in the special accommodation in which she lives. Instead, she has applied for and receives a home care grant: a grant that is given to Fadwa to compensate her for the care work she does despite not being formally hired by the special housing unit in which they now live. The young girl in question looks, in other words, after her grandmother around the clock and seldom goes out. This has implications for her social integration. She has studied Swedish but is now unemployed and receives maintenance support. The social worker who has granted both housing and the home care grant for her grandmother through HEC services is familiar with Fadwa's situation. She has advised Fadwa not to inform her colleague at IFC (the one that approved Fadwa's maintenance support) that she is the recipient of her grandmother's home care grant as well. Although this is probably a unique case, it is a good illustration of the problems that the division of social work practice into age-segregated units brings about. Particularly problematic is the fact that if it were revealed that Fadwa has withheld information about her income, she would risk not only losing her maintenance support but also being reported to the police. These are risks that the social worker who advised her to keep quiet about the arrangement must have been aware of. The ethical implications of this social worker's recommendations are, therefore, yet another angle to be considered. Equally interesting is the fact that this family seems to have a clear idea of what they will do once Fadwa marries and faces the demands of raising her own family. They are planning to arrange for her younger sister, who is not yet in Sweden, to migrate and takeover the care of their grandmother. This family could, in other words, become active in a transnational network for care (cf. Baldassar, 2007). Such networks have been shown to be of great importance to older migrants since they are considerably more adaptable to changing and specific needs, quicker to activate and are felt to be more neatly arranged than public, welfare state alternatives (Hillman, 2005). Irrespective of whether this family decides to address the care needs of the older woman through the activation of a transnational care network or not, the fact remains that this case clearly shows how migration is bringing about situations in which care work is performed in legal grey zones; grey zones that are in this country not only unregulated but also peripheral to welfare services at the moment. This example shows also that short-term solutions to current problems involving older migrants have the potential to set in motion transnational care solutions that could potentially challenge elder care in the long run.

Both of these cases show that social work practice with older people with migrant backgrounds can be more challenging than some seem to realise. They show also that there is an impending need to develop social work practice in order to meet both older migrants and their families' needs. Moreover, these cases show that the Swedish organisation of social work according to age groups (i.e., IFC and HEC) leads to different welfare actors' handling different aspects of the social position that being an ethnic 'Other' entails. As suggested earlier, in this country social work with younger individuals should ideally lead to work, integration and economic independence, while social work with older people focuses primarily on the provision of care. These two different ideals of social work practice should be kept in sight at all times since aiming for the latter with the older generation can jeopardise the former in the younger one. Of interest is also that this age-based division reflects the underlying ideal of individualism that is at the very core of the Swedish welfare state. The basic assumption is that young and old family members lead and want to lead separate lives, both financially and practically (Trägårdh & Berggren, 2006). The examples alluded to here show quite clearly that this ideal is being challenged by older migrants and their families. Social services that fail to see the generational implications of their decisions are in fact contributing to a situation in which different family members' needs can end up being regarded as competing needs. We cannot help but wonder whether the expectations we have on migrant families are compatible with the goal for greater social and economic integration of younger migrants who is at the core of Swedish social work practice.

In this respect it seems appropriate to ask what cutbacks in the Swedish welfare state will end up meaning for older migrants. There is a risk of greater culturalisation when resources are scarce since the equation of ethnic and cultural 'Otherness' with 'special needs' (as in the case of older migrants; cf. Torres, 2006) and with exceptional caring skills (as our own research suggests with respect to younger migrants working in elder care; cf. Torres, 2010a) could contribute to the implementation of parallel social work practices with unequal care quality controls. The situation that we are beginning to observe in Sweden suggests that older migrants are often cared for at home which means that they are being provided with care that risks being not only unregulated but also peripheral to mainstream social work practice. The cases alluded to here suggest also that the expectations on older migrant families are greater (cf. Forssell, 2004, 2010) than the expectations we seem to have on the families of older Swedes. There are, in other words, numerous risks for the ethnic 'Othering' of older migrants in Swedish social work and elder care and for relegating younger migrants to the periphery of society when they are encouraged to take on the role of informal caregivers for their elders. Hence, it seems appropriate to finish this article by quoting Warnes (2006) who has argued that:

> Migration must be conceived not as a single relocation decision by an individual at a moment in time, for this neglects important aspects of the formative and decision-making processes, and pays scant attention to the outcomes and consequences in both the short and the long terms. Migrations and later life need to be understood in their household, family and temporal contexts. As the main life-course stages have elaborated, and particularly the period of retirement has extended, a post-adolescent migrant's calculus must increasingly be influenced by his or her prospects and opportunities, not only during the second age but also through the third. (ibid, pp. 216–217)

It is because of this that we have argued that the development of gerontological social work practice in this country needs to not only become migration-aware but also generation-sensitive. Gerontological social work practice needs to also understand that the social position of ethnic 'Otherness' poses challenges to the very goals that the practice has set up for itself.

Acknowledgements

The authors wish to thank the Swedish Council for Working Life and Social Research for the support provided; the article has been written as part of a newly launched project titled 'Identifying needs in elderly clients with migrant backgrounds: are understandings of cross-cultural interaction, ethnic "Otherness" and gender relevant for need assessment practice?' (Dnr 2010-0666), which is lead by the second author. The first author wishes also to acknowledge the financial support received via the program grant titled 'Forms of care in later life: Agency, place, time and life course' awarded by the same funding organization to Prof. Eva Jeppsson Grassman (Dnr 2006-1621).

References

Ålund, A. & Schierup, C.-U. (1991) 'Prescribed multiculturalism in crisis', in *Paradoxes of Multiculturalism: Essays on Swedish Society*, eds A. Ålund & C.-U. Schierup, Avebury, Aldershot, pp. 1–20.

Andersson, K. (2007) 'Myndighetsutövning i äldreomsorgen: att skapa likhet i äldres behov' ['Excercising public authority in elderly care: creating similarities in the needs of elderly people'], in *Social omsorg i socialt arbete* [*Social Care in Social Work*], ed. S. Johansson, Gleerups, Malmö, pp. 152–172.

Baldassar, L. (2007) 'Transnational families and aged care: the mobility of care and the migrancy of ageing', *Journal of Ethnic and Migration Studies*, vol. 33, no. 2, pp. 275–297.

Bergmark, Å., Parker, M. C. & Thorslund, M. (2000) 'Priorities in care and services for elderly people: a path without guidelines?', *Journal of Medical Ethics*, vol. 26, pp. 312–318.

Blomberg, S. (2004) *Specialiserad biståndshandläggning inom den kommunala äldreomsorgen: genomförandet av en organisationsreform och dess praktik* [*Specialized Need Assessment within Municipal Elderly Care: Conducting an Organizational Reform and its Practice*], Ph.D. Dissertation, Lund University, Lund.

Blomberg, S., Edebalk, P. G. & Petersson, J. (2000) 'The withdrawal of the welfare state: elder care in Sweden in the 1990s', *European Journal of Social Work*, vol. 3, no. 2, pp. 151–163.

Bredström, A. (2002) 'Maskulinitet och kamp om nationella arenor: reflektioner kring bilden av "invandrarkillar" i svensk media' ['Masculinity and the struggle for national arenas: reflections on the image of migrant teenage boys in Swedish media'], in *Maktens (o)lika förklädnader: kön, klass och etnicitet i det postkoloniala Sverige* [*Power's Different Disguises: Gender, Class and Ethnicity in Post-Colonial Sweden*], eds P. de los Reyes, I. Molina & D. Mulinari, Atlas, Stockholm, pp. 182–206.

Brodin, H. (2005) *Does Anybody Care? Public and Private Responsibilities in Swedish Eldercare 1940–2000*, Dissertation, Umeå University.

Brune, Y. (2008) 'Bilden av invandrare i svenska nyhetsmedier' ['Images of ethnic 'Otherness' in Swedish news media'], in *Migration och etnicitet: perspektiv på ett mångkulturellt Sverige* [*Migration and Ethnicity: Perspectives on Multicultural Sweden*], eds M. Darvishpour & C. Westin, Studentlitteratur, Lund, pp. 335–361.

Cochrane, A., Clarke, J. & Gewirtz, S. (2001) *Comparing Welfare States*, SAGE, London.

Dunér, A. (2005) *Biståndshandläggningens villkor och dilemman inom äldre- och handikappomsorg* [*Need Assessment within Elderly and Disability Care: Conditions and Dilemmas*], Studentlitteratur, Lund.

Edström, N. (2008) *Socialt arbete i Botkyrka* [*Social Work in Botkyrka*], Botkyrka kommun och Mångkulturellt Centrum, Botkyrka.

Esping-Andersen, G. (1990) *The Three Worlds of Welfare Capitalism*, Polity Press, Cambridge.

Esping-Andersen, G. (1996) *Welfare States in Transition*, Sage, London.

Forssell, E. (2004) *Skyddandets förnuft. En studie om anhöriga till hjälpbehövande äldre som invandrat sent i livet* [*The Logic of Protection: A Study of Informal Caregiving to Older Family Members in Immigrant Families*], Ph.D. Dissertation, Stockholm University.

Forssell, E. (2006) 'Informell omsorg, socialt kapital och tillit' ['Informal care, social capital and trust'], in *Det civila samhället som forskningsfält: nya avhandlingar i ett nytt sekel: en antologi* [*Civic Society as a Research Field: New Dissertations in a New Century*], eds L. Svedberg & L. Trägårdh, Riksbankens Jubileumsfond och Gidlunds förlag, Hedemora, pp. 63–74.

Forssell, E. (2010) 'Anhörigomsorg i migrant familjer' ['Informal caregiving in migrant families'], in *Invandrarskap, äldrevård och omsorg* [*Ethnic 'Otherness' in Elder Care*], eds S. Torres & F. Magnússon, Gleerups, Malmö, pp. 93–105.

Gunnarsson, E. (2002) *Äldre utanför äldreomsorgen* [*Elderly in the Periphery of Elder Care*], National Board of Health and Welfare [Socialstyrelsen], Stockholm.

Heikkilä, K. (2004) *The Role of Ethnicity in Care of Elderly Finnish Immigrants*, Ph.D. Dissertation, Karolinska Institutet, Stockholm.

Heikkilä, K. (2010) 'Kulturanpassad äldrevård' ['Culture-sensitive elder care'], in *Invandrarskap, äldrevård och omsorg* [*Ethnic 'Otherness' in Elder Care*], eds S. Torres & F. Magnússon, Gleerups, Malmö, pp. 109–118.

Hillman, F. (2005) 'Migrants care work in private households, or the strength of bilocal and transnational ties as a last(ing) resource in global migration', in *Care and Social Integration in European Societies*, eds B. Pfau-Effinger & B. Geissler, Policy Press, Bristol, pp. 93–114.

Huset Mandag Morgen (2007) *What Lies Ahead for The Nordic model?: A Discussion Paper On The Future of The Nordic Welfare Model in A Global Competition Economy*, Nordic Council of Ministers [Norden], Copenhagen.

Janlöv, A.-C. (2006) *Participation in Needs Assessment of Older People prior to Public Home Help: Older Person's, their Family Members' and Assessing Home help Officers' Experiences*, Ph.D. Dissertation, Lund University, Lund.

Jegermalm, M. & Jeppsson Grassman, E. (2009a) 'Caregiving and volunteering among older people in Sweden: prevalence and profiles', *Journal of Aging and Social Policy*, vol. 21, pp. 352–373.

Jegermalm, M. & Jeppsson Grassman, E. (2009b) 'Patterns of informal help and caregiving in Sweden: a thirteen year perspective', *Social Policy and Administration*, vol. 43, no. 7, pp. 881–701.

Johansson, S. (ed.) (2007) *Social omsorg i socialt arbete* ['*Social Care in Social Work*'], Gleerups, Malmö.

Johansson, S. (ed.) (2010) *Omsorg och mångfald*, Gleerups, Malmö.

Kröger, T. (2005) 'Interplay between formal and informal care for older people: the state of the Nordic research', in *Äldreomsorgsforskning i Norden: en kunskapsöversikt* [*Nordic Elder Care Research: A Literature Review*], ed. M. Szebehely, TemaNord 2005: 508, Nordiska Ministerrådet, Köpenhamn.

Larsson, K. (2006) *Kvarboende eller flyttning på äldre dagar: en kunskapsöversikt* [*To Stay at Home or Move in Old Age: A Review of the Literature*], Stiftelsen Stockholms Läns Äldrecentrum, Stockholm.

Larsson, K. (2007) 'The social situation of older people', *International Journal of Social Welfare*, vol. 16, pp. 203–218.

Lindelöf, M. & Rönnbäck, E. (2004) *Att fördela bistånd: om handläggningsprocessen i äldreomsorgen* [*Approving Public Assistance: On the Need Assessment Process in Elderly Care*], Ph.D. Dissertation, Umeå University.

Machat, L. (2010) 'Bilden av "äldre invandrare" i äldrepolitiken' ['Images of older migrants in old age policy]', in *Invandrarskap, äldrevård och omsorg* [*Ethnic 'Otherness' in Elder Care*], eds S. Torres & F. Magnússon, Gleerups, Malmö, pp. 55–68.

Magnùsson, F. (ed.) (2007) *Drömmen om dagcentralen: omsorgsformer och språk bland utlandsfödda äldre i Malmö* [*The Dream of a Day-care Center: Care Types and Language Among Foreign-born Older People in Malmö*], Stadskontoret FoU-enheten/Kunskapsverkstaden 2007:2, Malmö.

Mattsson, K. (2001) 'Ekonomisk rasism: föreställningar om de Andra inom ekonomisk invandrarforskning' ['Economic rasism: understandings of ethnic 'Otherness' in economic migrant research]', in *Sverige och de Andra: postkoloniala perspektiv* [*Sweden and The 'Other': Post-Colonial Perspectives*], eds M. McEachrane & L. Faye, Natur och Kultur, pp. 243–264.

Olaison, A. (2009) *Negotiating Needs: Processing Older Persons as Home Help Care Recipients in Gerontological Social Work Practice*, Dissertation, Linköping University, Linköping Studies in Arts and Sciences No. 464.

Palme, J. Bergmark, Bäckman, O., Estrada, F., Fritzell, J., Lundberg, O., Sjöberg, O., Sommestad, L. & Szebehely, M. (2003) 'A welfare balance sheet for the 1990s: final report for the Swedish Welfare Commission', *Scandinavian Journal of Public Health, Supplement*, vol. 60, pp. 72–73.

Rauch, D. (2007) 'Is there really a Scandinavian social service model? A comparison of childcare and elder care in six European countries', *Acta Sociologica*, vol. 50, no. 3, pp. 249–269.

Regeringskansliet (2007) *Ministry of Health and Social Affairs Fact Sheet No. 18 (September 2007)*, Government Offices in Sweden [Regeringskansliet], Stockholm.

Ronström, O. (2002) 'The making of older immigrants in Sweden: identification, categorisation and discrimination', in *Cultural Gerontology*, ed. L. Andersson, Auburn House, Westport, CT.

Sand, A.-B. (2004) 'Förändrad tillämpning av offentlig äldreomsorg: ett hot mot målsättningen och demokrati och jämställdhet' ['Changed implementation of public elder care: a threat to the national goals, democracy and equality'], *Socialvetenskaplig tidskrift*, vol. 3–4, pp. 293–309.

Socialstyrelsen (2006) *Socialt arbete med äldre* [*Social Work with Older People*], National Board of Health and Welfare [Socialstyrelsen], Stockholm.

Socialstyrelsen (2009) *Vård och omsorg om äldre* [*Health and Social Care of Older People*], [*Socialstyrelsens lägesrapport 2008*] National Board of Health and Welfare, Stockholm.

Socialstyrelsen (2010) *Interkulturellt socialt arbete* [*Intercultural Social Work*], National Board of Health and Welfare [Socialstyrelsen], Stockholm.

Sundström, G. & Johansson, L. (2005) 'The changing balance of government and family care for the elderly in Sweden and other European countries'. *Australian Journal of Aging*, vol. 24 (suppl), pp. S5–S11.

Szebehely, M. (2000) 'Äldreomsorg i förändring: knappare resurser och nya organisationsformer' ['Elder care in the midst of change: fewer resources and new organisational forms'], in *Välfärd, vård och omsorg* [*Welfare and Care*], ed. M. Szebehely, Forskarantolog från Kommittén Välfärdsbokslutet, SOU 2000:38, Socialdepartamentet, Stockholm, pp. 171–224.

Szebehely, M. (ed.) (2003) *Hemhjälp i Norden: illustrationer och reflektioner* [*Home-help Care in Nordic Countries: Illustrations and Reflections*], Studentlitteratur, Lund.

Szebehely, M. (ed.) (2005) *Äldreomsorgsforskning i Norden: en kunskapsöversikt* [*Nordic Elder Care Research: A Literature Review*], TemaNord 2005: 508, Nordiska Ministerrådet, Köpenhamn.

Szebehely, M. & Trydegård, G.-B. (2007) 'Omsorgstjänster för äldre och funktionshindrade: skilda villkor, skilda trender?' ['Care services for elderly and disabled persons: different conditions, different trends'], *Socialvetenskaplig forskning*, vol. 2–3, pp. 197–219.

Szebehely, M. & Ullmanen, P. (2008) 'Vård av anhöriga: ett högt pris för kvinnor' ['Informal care: a high price to pay for women'], *Välfärd*, vol. 2, pp. 12–14.

Torres, S. (2006) 'Elderly Immigrants in Sweden: "Otherness" under construction', *Journal of Ethnic and Migration Studies*, vol. 32, no. 8, pp. 1341–1358.

Torres, S. (2008) 'The age of migration: what does it mean and why should European social gerontologists care?', in *Retraite et Sociéte* [Selection 2008], Caisse Nationale d'Assurance Viellesse, Paris, pp. 67–80.

Torres, S. (2010a) 'Invandrarskap och tvärkulturella äldreomsorgsmöten' ['Ethnic "Otherness" and cross-cultural elder care encounters'], in *Omsorg och mångfald* [Care and Diversity], ed. S. Johansson, Gleerups, Malmö, pp. 67–88.

Torres, S. (2010b) 'Inledning' ['Introduction'], in *Invandrarskap, äldrevård och omsorg* [*Ethnic 'Otherness' in Elder Care*], eds S. Torres & F. Magnússon, Gleerups, Malmö, pp. 9–16.

Torres, S. & Magnússon, F. (eds) (2010) *Invandrarskap, äldrevård och omsorg* [*Ethnic 'Otherness' in Elder Care*], Gleerups, Malmö.

Trydegård, G.-B. (2000) *Tradition, Change and Variation. Past and Present Trends in Public Old-age Care*, PhD dissertation, Stockholm University.

Trydegård, G.-B. & Thorslund, M. (2010) 'One uniform welfare state or a multitude of welfare municipalities? The evolution of local variation in Swedish elder care', *Social Policy and Administration*, vol. 44, no. 4, pp. 495–511.

Trägårdh, L. & Berggren, H. (2006) *Är svensken människa? Gemenskap och oberoende i det moderna Sverige* [*Are Swedes Humans? Community and Independence in Modern Sweden*], Norstedts, Sweden.

Warnes, A. M. (2006) 'The future life course, migration and the old age', in *The Futures of Old Age*, eds J. A. Vincent, C. R. Phillipson & M. Downs, Sage, London, pp. 208–217.

The experiences and expectations of care and support among older migrants in the UK

Gianfranco Giuntoli & Mima Cattan

This paper reports and critically discusses, against the literature on culturally sensitive and cultural competency practices, the findings of a qualitative study which explored the needs and expectations of older people and their carers from eight different migrant communities and the white British majority. The study investigated the accessibility and acceptability of care and support services in Bradford, UK, a city with a large migrant population. A total of 167 study participants were recruited from February 2008 to October 2008; of these 134 were older people and 33 carers. The age ranged from 25 to 90 years. The study found that older migrants and their carers described expectations of services as complex constructions of 'abstract expectations', the study participants' general beliefs regarding what services should be about, and 'pragmatic expectations', their specific views about how they would like to receive care and access services. All groups, irrespective of their ethnic background, expressed three 'abstract expectations': high standards of good practice; cultural understanding; and responsiveness to individual expectations. This similarity did not imply a similarity in their preferences for how services should provide for their 'abstract expectations'. Dignity was a central expectation for all older people in the care of their bodies. However, a number of culturally specific 'pragmatic expectations' emerged in the practices that older people and carers associated with maintaining dignity in older age. Nevertheless, differences could not always be explained as an outcome of different cultural backgrounds, but were rather linked to individual characteristics and life experiences. This study indicates that whether and how older migrants' knowledge systems inform their expectations of care and support should be objects of investigation rather than taken for granted, as implied in some literature on culturally sensitive practices. Exploration of older migrants' knowledge systems may help us to understand if older migrants' expectations differ with regard to what they expect to receive from a certain service, their 'abstract expectations', and/or how they expect to receive it, their 'pragmatic expectations'. This information should help to identify if different communities require different culturally competent interventions and of what type: interventions at the organisational level, at the structural level or at the clinical level.

Introduction

In recent years, research has shown a rapid growth in the number of migrants ageing in Europe, with higher rates of increase in the middle-old and oldest-old age groups (Fenton, 1987; Blakemore, 1999, 2000; White, 2006). Despite some variations in countries and migrant communities (White, 2006), this phenomenon is common to the five types of older international migrants identified in the literature: older forced migrants, European labour migrants, older non-European migrants, older family joiners and returning post-retirement migrants (Warnes *et al.*, 2004; Dwyer & Papadimitriou, 2006). This rapid increase in older people is mirrored across European populations (de Groot *et al.*, 2004), due to longer life expectancy combined with a decline in birth rates. These demographic changes have important implications for health and social care sectors and create new requirements for the facilitation of social inclusion and access to public services across Europe (Warnes *et al.*, 2004; Messkoub, 2005; Dwyer & Papadimitriou, 2006).

Since the 1980s, social work theory has increasingly emphasised the significance of culturally sensitive practices for services to meet the needs of users from different cultural backgrounds (among others, Devore & Schlesinger, 1981; Graham, 1999; Schiele, 2000; Sue, 2003; Yu, 2006, 2009). This approach criticises the dominance of the Eurocentric worldview in social work and attempts to develop practice on the basis of other cultural groups' knowledge systems, for example African worldviews regarding the interconnectedness of all things (Graham, 1999; Schiele, 2000), Confucian principles such as ren (Yu, 2000), and the five pillars of Islam (Dean & Khan, 1997).

Different authors have referred to culturally sensitive practices using different expressions, for example cultural sensitivity, cultural competence, cross-cultural expertise, cultural awareness and cultural responsiveness, with cultural sensitivity and cultural competence the most popular terms (Whaley, 2008). In an examination of the semantic relationship between the terms cultural sensitivity and cultural competence Whaley (2008) demonstrated that the two expressions are at opposite ends of a common dimension. Cultural sensitivity refers to clinicians' awareness and knowledge of different cultural beliefs, traditions and behaviours, whereas cultural competence refers to the specific skills and knowledge of the techniques that can be useful to act competently with a culturally diverse clientele (Whaley, 2008). The results of Whaley's (2008) analyses are consistent with other authors' argument that awareness and knowledge of different cultural traditions are necessary but not sufficient to provide culturally competent services (Brach & Fraser, 2000). Cultural competency in service provision implies moving beyond the promotion of cultural awareness or sensitivity towards an 'ongoing commitment or institutionalisation of appropriate practice and policies for diverse populations' (Brach & Fraser, 2000, p. 183). Awareness, knowledge and skills are critical elements of cultural competency in social work as well (Yan & Wong, 2005). However, in addition, Yan and Wong (2005) emphasise the relevance of social workers' self-awareness of their own cultural background for the effectiveness of cultural competency practises.

Despite the growing popularity of the concepts of cultural sensitivity and cultural competence and the development of cultural competency guidelines and policies, especially in the United States (National Association of Social Workers, 2001; US Department of Health and Human Services Office of Minority Health, 2001), these concepts have been criticised on several grounds. Some authors have criticised the lack of rigorous research evaluating the impact of cultural competency techniques on any outcomes, including the reduction of racial and ethnic disparities (Brach & Fraser, 2000). Others have criticised the unevaluated assumptions that often characterise these approaches, particularly the assumption that older migrants' expectations are both strongly and consistently culturally characterised (Gross, 1995; Simon & Mosavel, 2008; Yu, 2009). Yu (2009) points out that the literature on culturally sensitive practices is often underpinned by two beliefs; that 'all members of the same ethnic minority group organise their health and social care according to their cultural principles' (p. 57), and that older migrants' 'cultural principles are monolithic' (p. 57). These assumptions imply that older migrants tend to have different expectations of care and support services compared to the indigenous, national majorities. However, there is scant research on these assumptions (Simon & Mosavel, 2008). Most of the literature on cultural competency models has discussed the models from two perspectives. Firstly, there are the criticisms of the view that 'culture' and 'ethnic background' are the most important factors to address in order to tackle health inequalities in multicultural societies. Blacksher (2008) and Simon and Mosavel (2008) demonstrate the complimentary and at times stronger saliency of class and socio-economic status to understand health inequalities. Wimmer (2009) discusses the importance of not taking the concepts of ethnicity and culture as 'unproblematic *explanans*' in migrant studies; in other words, as self-evident units of observation and analysis. He refers to the boundary-making paradigm and shows how this approach considers ethnicity as an '*explanandum*, i.e. as a variable outcome of specific processes to be analytically uncovered and empirically specified' (p. 244). Secondly, there is critique that focuses on the limits of the classic anthropological view of culture, which underpins most cultural competency models. In this view, culture is conceptualised as an organic and separate whole of values, customs and beliefs, etc. for which it is possible to clearly define what is 'inside' and what is 'outside' (Simon & Mosavel, 2008). Dean (2001) and Yan and Wong (2005), who draw on constructivist and postmodern perspectives, suggest that cultural expectations are constantly re-constructed and re-negotiated by immigrants according to their changing life circumstances. Consequently, they cannot be conceptualised as stable and unchangeable sets of values and norms. Other authors have investigated elderly care practices in different migrant communities and shown that in many cases cultural principles are not monolithic but change over time to adapt to the migrants' life circumstances (Chiu & Yu, 2001; Lan, 2002; Ajrouch, 2005). However, these studies have focused on the investigation of traditional values and practices of single migrant groups and on the relevance of such values for the development of culturally sensitive practices for these groups. Little is known regarding why and how differences and similarities arise across groups of older migrants and between older migrants and national majorities, and to what extent older migrants' expectations and use of services differ in their everyday life from those of national majorities.

The purpose of this article is to explore these latter issues and their relevance for culturally sensitive practices. It does so by describing and discussing the findings from a study which set out to explore commonalities and differences in care and support needs and expectations and in the perceptions of accessibility and acceptability of care and support within and between older migrant groups and national majorities. The study was conducted in Bradford, a northern city in England, UK, with a high proportion of migrant groups.

Background

In the UK, the population aged 65 and over currently accounts for 16% of the total population and, in line with the rest of Europe, is predicted to continue rising. The fastest increases in numbers is in the 'oldest old' group, those aged 85 years and over, who represent over 2% of the population (Dunnell, 2008). By 2020, it is estimated that ethnic minority people will comprise 5% of the 60-plus population, compared with about 1.7% in 1991 (Grewal et al., 2004). As a result, increasing government policy attention has been given to the implications of an ageing population for future services for older people (see for example Department of Health, 2001, 2006, 2007; Social Exclusion Unit, 2006).

Several local initiatives, including in Bradford (Bradford Metropolitan Council, 2007), have also been launched. However, in a review, Darlow et al. (2005) noted a general lack of research on issues of social care in Bradford. The report criticised existing research for being too focused on specific migrant groups (Pakistani, Bangladeshi and Indian) to the exclusion or under-representation of others, particularly migrant groups of white European background (Chahal & Temple, 2005; Darlow et al. 2005). It suggested that there was a need for further in-depth research in this field, taking into account the individual needs of elders and carers in different migrant groups at local level. Indeed, one of the difficulties for service providers in Bradford has been the uncertainty of not fully understanding the experiences, needs and preferences of older people and their carers with regards to health, social welfare and other services (Outside Research and Development, 2006).

Methods

The study involved older people and carers (the term 'carer' is used throughout this article and has the same meaning as 'caregiver' in the US literature) from eight migrant communities and the white British majority. The eight migrant communities were: Polish, Ukrainian, Italian, Hungarian, Pakistani, Indian, Bangladeshi and Afro Caribbean. The research had two distinct stages: a literature review and the data collection, analysis and synthesis. A total of 134 older people and 33 carers were recruited and interviewed from February 2008 to October 2008; 126 were females (75.45%) and 41 were males (24.55%). Older age was defined as being above 60 years of age for women and above 65 years of age for men. However, some study participants, predominantly men of South Asian background (Pakistani, Bangladeshi and Indians), self-identified themselves as 'old' although they were not above 65 years of age. Tables 1 and 2 provide a breakdown of the study participants by ethic group and age.

Older people and carers were approached through gatekeepers of a range of community groups and organisations, for example mosques, working men's clubs and carers' organisations. Each organisation was provided with written information about the project, including posters or newsletters in appropriate languages. The recruitment aimed to include older people and carers who were service users at the time of the interview, who were not service users at the time of the interview, but had been in the past, and who had never accessed care or support services at the time of the interview. Only a minority of the participants had previously participated in evaluations of specific services.

The data collection consisted of two phases. In the first phase a total of 21 focus groups were carried out, of which 12 focus groups were with older migrants and five focus groups were with their carers. The focus groups varied in size from 3 to 21 study participants. In the second phase, 53 in-depth interviews with 38 older people and 15 carers were undertaken. Participants were partly identified through the focus groups and partly newly recruited on the basis of their self-reported care needs and current or past experiences of social care services.

Table 1 Breakdown of the study participants by ethnic group

Ethnic group	N	%
White British	37	22.16
Pakistani	34	20.36
Italian	21	12.57
Bangladeshi	19	11.38
Polish	15	8.98
Indian	13	7.78
Ukrainian	12	7.19
Hungarian	9	5.39
African Caribbean	7	4.19
Totals	167	100

Table 2 Breakdown of study participants by age group

Age groups	N	%
25–35	5	2.99
36–45	7	4.19
46–59	21	12.57
60–65	14	8.38
66–70	40	23.95
71–75	27	16.17
76–80	26	15.57
81–90	22	13.17
Missing values	5	2.99
Totals	167	100

The focus group interview schedules explored the extent to which older people and their carers considered that their care and support needs were, or might be, met and by whom. After piloting the interview schedule, case studies in the form of vignettes were developed to stimulate discussion and to ensure understanding and articulation of the issues being explored in the focus group interview. These were well received by the study participants as they enabled them to contribute to the discussion without necessarily disclosing personal experiences. We also found that older people were more likely to express their personal needs and desires if hypothetical cases based on familiar situations were presented to them than if they were asked to consider something that seemed more abstract. The focus group interviews provided an opportunity for participating older people and carers to get to know and trust the research team, which helped in the exploration of personal and often sensitive experiences in the in-depth interviews.

The purpose of the in-depth interviews was to give interviewees an opportunity to talk through their lives (narrative approach), while reflecting on their contacts with and experiences of a range of services, such as health, community support, social care or housing. This enabled exploration of the 'caring period' as well as the transitional time preceding caring for/being cared for. In some cases, older people's experiences related to experiences outside the UK and helped to ground perceptions of current services, needs and aspirations within their cultural framework.

Sixteen interpreters were involved in the study to assist those study participants who were not fluent in or did not speak English. The interpreters were recruited through the Bradford Interpreting Unit for the following languages: Urdu, Gujarati, Punjabi, Bangla, Hungarian, Polish, Ukrainian and Italian. To ensure that the research team and the interpreters shared a common understanding of research practice, roles and responsibilities, needs and expectations, a two-day training event was organised before the interviews commenced. The training event provided an opportunity to explore the interpreters' beliefs and expectations about their role, the research and the research team. Most interpreters embraced a positivist view regarding their role. They saw themselves as neutral in the interview process and thought that the meanings of the study participants' answers could be reported unambiguously. In order to stimulate self-awareness among the interpreters, the research team presented a number of exercises based on ad hoc case studies. The aim was to encourage discussion among the interpreters about what the 'right' translation of a number of controversial extracts from imaginary conversations was. These exercises highlighted how important it was for the interpreters to discuss with the research team any difficulties they experienced in the translation process.

In each interview session, the interpreters were required to translate the interview questions from English to the relevant language and the interviewees' answers from the relevant language into English. This gave little time to consider problems in their translations. To ease this task the interpreters were asked to comment on the interview schedule of both the focus groups and the individual interviews. These discussions highlighted some potential issues concerning the translation of certain words, for example 'carers', in particular languages. Consequently, the training and the ensuing discussions helped to improve the clarity of the interview schedules and to strengthen the inclusion of the interpreters in the interview process.

All the interviews were conducted by the first author and transcribed verbatim by a professional service. The analysis of the focus group interviews was based on 'Framework Analysis' (Ritchie & Lewis, 2003), which is framed around five recursive phases: construction of an *indexing or coding table* based on issues and questions derived from the literature review, aims and objectives of the study, and recurring views and experiences of the study participants; *indexing or coding* the data, where the thematic framework is applied systematically to the raw data; *charting*, where a number of charts representing key themes identified through the indexing process are created, and the data sorted by means of distilled summaries of the participants' views and experiences; *mapping and interpretation*, where the summaries in each chart are used to find associations between themes to provide explanations for the findings.

The analysis of the in-depth interviews was informed by a narrative approach. Here the interviewee tells a story, thereby constructing a social reality which is 'meaningful' (Elliott, 2005). The analysis needs to be theoretical, in that themes are drawn from the interviewees' realities of the social and cultural world. The analysis is not simply about 'what' people say but also about 'how' they express their experiences, desires and expectations. This process of analysis is particularly suited for qualitative research where it is likely that those involved have different life experiences and social realities. A systematic approach to analyse the study participants' narratives in order to discover the patterns, regularities and meaning-making processes within their interviews was devised based on Franzosi (1994, 2004). In this approach the subject, the action and the social actors mentioned by the study participants are first defined. This is followed by examining in detail the social actors (in this case those involved in help and support) and the action (here the action of receiving help and support).

The electronic qualitative software package Nvivo 7.0 (QSR International, 2007) was used to organise, code the data and assist with its analysis. The data was coded and analysed by the first author. In addition, for validity purposes, a sample of the interviews was coded by the second author and the codings compared to identify and discuss any possible disagreement.

The combined synthesis of the focus group interviews and the narrative interviews led to the identification of common themes in the study participants' experiences of care and support and to the identification of their expectations regarding the accessibility and acceptability of services.

Ethical approval for the study was obtained from the Faculty Research Ethics Committee at Leeds Metropolitan University. All participants in the interviews were given an information sheet detailing the project and their rights to withdraw from it at any time. In order to make sure that the study participants felt comfortable with the interpreters who were assigned to them, the name and photo of the interpreters were printed in the information leaflets. This gave the study participants opportunity to contact the research team if they knew the interpreter and felt that this could jeopardise the confidentiality of their interview. Each participant provided written consent to participate in the study prior to the interview. All interviews were conducted in a familiar location, such as a community centre and were tape recorded with the interviewees' consent.

Findings

The analysis of the focus groups and individual interviews showed that the study participants' views about caring relationships and access to services were linked and complex and could be heuristically divided into two components:

(1) 'Abstract expectations', which referred to the study participants' general views regarding what an accessible and acceptable service should consist of (e.g. respect for dignity, high professional standard and communication). Irrespective of their ethnic background, the study participants shared the following abstract expectations: that emotional needs such as communication, trust, dignity and relief from loneliness were met to achieve a satisfactory and long lasting caring relationship and that services delivered 'high standards of good practice'.

(2) 'Pragmatic expectations' which consisted of the specific meaning that each 'abstract expectation' held for older migrants and their carers. 'Pragmatic expectations' consisted of older migrants' and their carers' views of what precisely was important to maintain dignity in older age, which issues were important in the caring communication, and what professional practices were particularly sensitive.

These two types of expectations are presented under the following two main themes: emotional needs and access to services needs, which are based on Helgeson's (2003) classification of support. These needs refer to people's experiences of the availability of people who can listen, care, sympathise and make one feel valued and loved, and the provision of information or guidance.

Emotional needs

Participants' experiences of help and support were often strongly linked to emotional needs, based on psychological factors, feelings and wishes, with communication, trust, dignity and relief from loneliness identified as particularly important for participants. The importance of these emotional needs was consistent across all the ethnic groups involved in the study, suggesting that the participants shared common 'abstract expectations' regarding how their emotional needs were met. However, with regards to their 'pragmatic expectations' about how services should address older people's emotional needs differences arose mainly around the issues of communication and dignity but not regarding trust and relief from loneliness.

Communication

When participants talked about communication, they described the need for an ongoing dialogue within and between services, between services and service recipients and between the carer and the person needing care about individual preferences, needs and entitlements, for example:

> When my mum first came out [of the hospital] they assessed her. She was wheel chair bound, they said oh don't worry we will get a ramp up. They sent some builders up within three, four weeks of mum coming out of hospital and we had this construction in the back yard. I looked at it and thought, one it's in the backyard, two it looks like you can launch a space rocket off this thing [...] Mum was already apprehensive about being in a wheel chair never mind being pushed four foot in the air, totally unacceptable [...] So the assessment was done, they ticked their boxes when they provided the ramp, but they didn't mention that it was access to the back [...] Well common sense would have told you to have some kind of discussion with the client, that seldom never happens. (Male Afro Caribbean British carer, 46)

Both carers and older people considered it crucial to address communication issues at group/community/cohort level as well as at the individual, face to face level of the caring relationship:

> If I gave her a meal on Tuesday and she ate it, it would be oh she likes that I will give her that Wednesday, Thursday, Friday. But come Wednesday and it's like: 'what's wrong? I thought you liked that?' 'But you can't give it to me everyday!' Now I tell her what's available and it makes my life a lot easier [...] I think it is just [a matter of] understanding and compassion and communication. I think that if you have those three things you get on with anybody you have to care for. (Male Afro Caribbean British carer, 46)

At the group or cohort level, the study participants' cultural and spiritual backgrounds played a critical role in determining the specific issues that they considered important in the communication process. Although all study participants shared a common 'abstract expectation' regarding the role of communication in the caring process, the specific issues, their 'pragmatic expectations', differed from group to group. For example, white British older carers suggested that their parents' generation often did not like to receive help from non-family members, and argued that these attitudes and expectations had to be recognised when planning and providing care and support for this cohort of much older people:

> My mother was like that, she didn't want any strangers come in at all, she didn't even want the carers [...] My dad was ill and he had to have the nurse three times a day to see him and she didn't even want them. It right upset her. I used to have to stop at night until they came so that she could go to bed before they came [...] My mother's age group were all sort of family things like that and they didn't go out that much. Our generation mix more, so you might have in years to come like us we won't do that. (White British older woman, 68, living with husband)

Polish carers commented that their parents' experience of never having cared for their own ageing parents, as they were left in Poland, together with their experiences of occupation and deportation during the Second World War, had shaped their expectations of care and support in old age in two ways. Firstly, their parents expected to receive support and company from their children at all times during the day. Secondly, their parents did not want any external help, as they had often developed a strong fear of 'officers' as a consequence of their experiences during the Second World War:

> My mum doesn't want any external help. If there were two of me and one could be with mum all the time and the other person who does their own thing all the time that would be great, but mum only wants me. (Polish carer, 56, living with husband)

> When the mail came and my parents saw a brown envelope they used to be terrified because they thought 'who is it?' My mother, even today, she is eighty three, she thinks that at some point they are going to be sending her back to Poland and she has nowhere to go, as her village no longer exists. They are frightened of bureaucracy; assessments on them to see what they have got, how are they going to manage, it smacks of bureaucracy.... (Polish carer, 54, living with husband and mother)

Another common 'pragmatic expectation' concerning communication was related to older people's need for increased time to process information, which had a major impact on face-to-face interactions with care staff, such as assessments. Many interviewees suggested that social workers should allow more time for older people to process the information and to share it with their next of kin, as illustrated by these quotes:

> When professional carers say to older people, regardless of what nationality they are, 'Do you understand?' I think they should err on the side of caution, because older people can have dementia or a bit of Alzheimer's and when they say 'yes' today, tomorrow it means 'no' [...] I object to social workers talking to my mum when I am not present, because I know that my mother would say things to please

them, but she is not telling them the truth. (Polish carer, 54, living with husband and mother)

For older migrants who were not fluent in or able to speak English access to interpreters was also linked to effective communication. The removal of language barriers was often the first step towards trust and a greater understanding between the older migrant and those who provided services.

Trust

The issue of trust was mainly raised in two ways: trusting care staff and personal safety. Several older people mentioned that they had to have confidence in their care staff before they could trust them with those tasks that were important to their quality of life, but which they could no longer do themselves. Trust took time to develop, but the presence of some form of previous connection between the older person and the care worker facilitated the development of trust. Importantly, these connections did not necessarily imply a common ethnic background between the carer and the older person:

> There was a black carer who came here and she realised that I was good friends with her brother and that level of trust actually built, I was reliant on her, mum developed a relationship and loved it. Then there was a white carer who came in and I actually went to school with her and she was now caring and it was a case of well I know you from school and mum developed really good relationships with them [. . .]. (Male Afro Caribbean British carer, 46)

For many interviewees, having 'strangers' visiting them raised issues of personal safety. Although none of the people we interviewed had felt threatened by their care staff, they worried that they might be deceived or robbed. Older people and their carers, regardless of their ethnic background, had common 'pragmatic expectations' regarding the factors that could help to build and maintain trust in caring relationships. These included having meetings between older people and care staff preceding the start of care services to get to know one another, consistency in the care staff who made home visits, and appropriate information regarding the time of visits and identity of the care workers.

Dignity

Dignity was described as having a caring relationship based on respect. In other words, they expected to be listened to and taken seriously, and as one Bangladeshi woman said: 'not being hurt in any way'. Dignity, therefore, meant that both their bodies and their feelings were respected.

Dignity was a common 'abstract expectation' for all older people in the care relationship. However, their 'pragmatic expectations' emerged in the practices that older people and carers associated with maintaining dignity in older age. Some differences were evidently related to older people's and carers' specific cultural backgrounds. For example, for Afro Caribbean older migrants, dignity in the care of their bodies meant having their bodies moisturised on a regular basis in a culturally responsive manner, a factor which did not appear in other groups. For Pakistani and Bangladeshi older migrants their religious identity as Muslims was a strong guiding factor in their expectations of care. A critical factor for them was, therefore, to have care staff of the same sex. For white British older people, the ability to maintain independence was a central, strong issue associated with dignity. However, some differences were also related to specific individual idiosyncrasies. For example, for some white British older people the question of dignity was also associated with the ability to maintain their house to a certain standard of tidiness:

> When a person has been house proud all their life and they sit there and they're looking round their home and they're thinking 'oh that wants doing' if they can't get jobs done that they used to do, that could do more damage to their health than anything else. (White British woman, 82, former home carer)

Relief from loneliness

Loneliness was consistently described as spending long periods of time in solitude without talking to or having meaningful social interaction with anyone. It often seemed to be the final outcome of a process of loss, one after the other, of valued companions until the point when no companionship was perceived as available. Missing the contact with close family members, such as partners, sons and daughters, was frequently the first element in the participants' descriptions of loneliness. Older migrants often described the unavailability of members of their own community of origin with whom to interact socially as a significant loss.

Most of the suggestions for ways to relieve loneliness were based on older participants' 'pragmatic expectations' of what might alleviate loneliness in later life. Some suggested visits to day centres or community centres as ways to ease older people's loneliness:

> The day centre where my husband goes all day Monday, Thursday and Friday morning. Today they are out for the day trip. That is the best thing [speaking of how to ease loneliness]. (White British woman, 83, living with visually impaired husband)

> They know a woman who now attends the centre and who they knew was used to spend long periods of time alone, feeling lonely. So, they invited her to come to the centre and spend time with them [referring to group of woman attending focus group]. So she started to come and she felt a lot better. (Focus group with Bangladeshi older women, through interpreter)

Access to services needs

Participants expressed strong views about what constituted 'good practice' in the way services were delivered. This expectation was related to the needs of trust and communication discussed previously and had a major impact on decisions about retaining services or not. The notion of 'good practice' was associated with perceptions of professional and ethical standards in the delivery of services.

Examples of perceived poor professional and ethical practices included:

(1) Care staff not washing their hands on arrival, for each new client;
(2) Using the same cloth to wash the older person's face as well as the rest of their body;
(3) Not following basic hygiene practices such as cleaning the bowl used to wash the older person and re-using it dirty the following day;
(4) Not tidying up after completion of care tasks;
(5) Not respecting the dignity of the individual.

There were similarities between study participants in their request for high standards of good practice, their 'abstract expectation', and mostly in the specific issues that were considered as important elements of good practice, their 'pragmatic expectations'. However, some older migrants and carers stressed the relevance of specific practices within their culture. For example, African Caribbean carers stressed the importance of hygiene in their culture:

> When my mother had her car accident [...] we had home care coming, but I had to keep an eye on what homecare were doing, how we care for ourselves is not how the English would take care [...]. (Female Afro Caribbean British carer, 34, living with family)

Pakistani and Bangladeshi study participants stressed the importance of their identity as Muslims. In their words, it was important to acknowledge the practices and behaviours related to their religion in service provision, for example, halal food, same sex care staff and prayer rooms in housing services. However, some older Bangladeshi women said that they did not expect care staff to replicate all behaviours associated with cultural or religious beliefs, such as feeding with the hand. They simply expected that staff talked to the older people about their desires, that the tasks were executed properly whilst at the same time respecting older people's dignity.

Discussion

This study set out to investigate the needs, experiences and aspirations of care and support among older people and carers from a range of migrant and white British communities across Bradford in the UK. Ideas for the development of culturally sensitive services were also explored. Our findings showed that, despite different experiences and cultural backgrounds, the study participants shared a number of common 'abstract expectations'. Most differences in the study participants' views emerged at the level of their 'pragmatic expectations'. Interestingly, these differences could not always be explained as an outcome of different cultural backgrounds, but were rather linked to individual characteristics and life experiences.

The literature on older migrants' needs of care and support and on culturally sensitive practices in health and social care services emphasises the importance for professionals and policy-makers to acknowledge the wider cultural expectations, and the individual expectations of older migrants and their carers. However, to date there is a lack of understanding of the interaction between culturally based expectations and individual expectations and of how the views of care and support and access to services across different groups of older migrants and between older migrants and national majorities are shaped. This lack of a theoretical framework has often resulted in an over-emphasis of the importance of cultural factors or of individual differences, whilst ignoring the interaction between them. This study identified two distinct types of expectations in older people's views of care and support services: 'abstract expectations' and 'pragmatic expectations'. Our analysis has shown that, despite their different backgrounds, the study participants had a significant element of similarity in that they shared a number of common 'abstract expectations'.

Although our study did not identify significant differences with regards to older migrants' 'abstract expectations' of the issues investigated, it does not necessarily imply that all older people share one common cultural knowledge system. However, the similarities found at the level of 'abstract expectations' support Yu's (2009) conclusion that researchers cannot take for granted that older migrants' expectations are necessarily informed by a different and monolithic cultural knowledge system. If and how older migrants' different knowledge systems inform their expectations should be objects of investigation rather than taken for granted. Taking the example of loneliness, the solutions suggested by the interviewees were based on their knowledge of available services rather than on cultural expectations. However, currently there is insufficient evidence to demonstrate if there are cultural or ethnic differences in the factors that impact on loneliness or in the interventions that might prevent or alleviate loneliness in later life (Cattan *et al.*, 2005; Victor *et al.*, 2005).

Exploration of older migrants' knowledge systems may help us to understand if older migrants' expectations differ with regard to *what* they expect to receive from a certain service, their 'abstract expectations', and/or *how* they expect to receive it, in other words their 'pragmatic expectations'. This information should help to identify if different communities require different culturally competent interventions and of what type: interventions at the organisational level, e.g. more representativeness, at the structural level, e.g. interpreter services, or at the clinical level, e.g. training interventions for care providers.

Our findings have shown some of the complexities of the cognitive and meaning-making processes that form older migrants' expectations of care and support. The two types of expectations that were identified through the analysis have allowed us to identify a continuum of similarities and differences in older people's expectations. However, our study only focused on one limited area of influences on older people's service expectations. There is, therefore, still need for theoretical frameworks that would help to disentangle ethnic processes from non-ethnic processes in the interpretations. The concepts suggested in this article and Wimmer's (2009) suggestions regarding how migrants' experiences and actions should be accounted for without a priori assuming ethnicity as an *explanans* can help researchers to investigate how and why diversity and similarity arise across and within migrant groups.

Acknowledgements

This study was funded by the Joseph Rowntree Foundation as part of an ongoing commitment to the development of services in Bradford.

References

Ajrouch, K. J. (2005) 'Arab-American immigrant elders' views about social support', *Ageing & Society*, vol. 25, no. 5, pp. 655–673.

Blacksher, E. (2008) 'Healthcare disparities: the salience of social class', *Cambridge Quarterly of Healthcare Ethics*, vol. 17, no. 2, pp. 143–153.

Blakemore, K. (1999) 'International migration in later life: social care and policy implications', *Ageing and Society*, vol. 16, pp. 761–774.

Blakemore, K. (2000) 'Health and social care needs in minority communities: an over-problematised issue?', *Health and Social Care in the Community*, vol. 8, pp. 22–30.

Brach, C. & Fraser, I. (2000) 'Can cultural competency reduce racial and ethnic health disparities? A review and conceptual model', *Medical Care Research and Review*, vol. 57, Suppl. 1, pp. 181–217.

Bradford Metropolitan Council (2007) *Older People*, Bradford City Council, Bradford.

Cattan, M., White, M., Bond, J. & Learmouth, A. (2005) 'Preventing social isolation and loneliness among older people: a systematic review of health promotion interventions', *Ageing and Society*, vol. 25, no. 1, pp. 41–67.

Chahal, K. & Temple, B. (2005) 'A review of research on minority ethnic older people', *SAGE Race Relations Abstracts*, vol. 30, no. 4, pp. 3–40.

Chiu, S. & Yu, S. (2001) 'An excess of culture: the myth of shared care in the Chinese community in Britain', *Ageing and Society*, vol. 21, no. 6, pp. 681–699.

Darlow, A., Bickerstaffe, T., Burden, T., Green, J., Jassi, S., Johnson, S., Kelsey, S., Purcell, M., South, J. & Walton, F. (2005) *Researching Bradford*, Leeds Metropolitan University, New York.

Dean, R. G. (2001) 'The myth of cross-cultural competence', *Families in Society*, vol. 82, no. 6, pp. 623–630.

Dean, H. & Khan, Z. (1997) 'Muslim perspectives on welfare', *Journal of Social Policy*, vol. 26, no. 2, pp. 193–209.

de Groot, L. C. P. M. G., Verheijden, M. W., de Henauw, S., Schroll, M., van Staveren, W. A. & Seneca Investigators (2004) 'Lifestyle, nutritional status, health, and mortality in elderly people across Europe: a review of the longitudinal results of the SENECA study', *Journals of Gerontology Series A—Biological Sciences and Medical Sciences*, vol. 59, pp. 1277–1284.

Department of Health (2001) *National Service Framework for Older People*, Department of Health, London.

Department of Health (2006) *Our Health, Our Care, Our Say: A New Direction For Community Services*, The Stationary Office, London.

Department of Health (2007) *Putting People First: A Shared Vision and Commitment to the Transformation of Adult Social Care*, Department of Health, London.

Devore, W. & Schlesinger, E. G. (1981) *Ethnic-Sensitive Social Work Practice*, C.V. Mosby Co, St. Louis, MO.

Dunnell, K. (2008) *Ageing and Mortality in the UK: Population Trends*, Office for National Statistics, Basingstoke.

Dwyer, P. & Papadimitriou, D. (2006) 'The social security rights of older international migrants in the European Union', *Journal of Ethnic and Migration Studies*, vol. 32, pp. 1301–1319.

Elliott, J. (2005) *Using Narrative in Social Research. Qualitative and Quantitative Approaches*, Sage, London.

Fenton, S. (1987) *Ageing Minorities: Black People as They Grow Old in Britain*, Commission for Racial Equality, London.

Franzosi, R. (1994) 'From words to numbers: a set theory framework for the collection, organization, and analysis of narrative data', *Sociological Methodology*, vol. 24, pp. 105–136.

Franzosi, R. (2004) *From Words to Numbers: Narrative, Data, and Social Science*, Cambridge University Press, Cambridge.

Graham, M. (1999) 'The African-centred worldview: developing a paradigm for social work', *British Journal of Social Work*, vol. 29, no. 2, pp. 252–267.

Grewal, I., Nazroo, J., Bajekal, M., Blane, D. & Lewis, J. (2004) 'Influences on quality of life: a qualitative investigation of ethnic differences among older people in England', *Journal of Ethnic & Migration Studies*, vol. 30, no. 4, pp. 737–761.

Gross, E. R. (1995) 'Deconstructing politically correct practice literature: the American Indian case', *Social Work*, vol. 40, no. 2, pp. 206–213.

Helgeson, V. S. (2003) 'Social support and quality of life', *Quality of Life Research*, vol. 12, pp. 25–31.

Lan, P. (2002) 'Subcontracting filial piety', *Journal of Family Issues*, vol. 23, pp. 812–835.

Messkoub, M. (2005) 'Migrants in the European Union: welfare in old age' *Public Finance & Management*, vol. 5, pp. 269–289.

National Association of Social Workers (2001) *NASW Standards For Cultural Competence in Social Work Practice*, NASW Press, Washington, DC.

Outside Research and Development (2006) *Care Needs of Older People in Manningham*, Outside Research and Development, Leeds.

QSR International (2007) NVivo 7, [Online] Available at: http://www.qsrinternational.com/ (accessed 24 Sept. 2009).

Ritchie, J. & Lewis, J. (eds) (2003) *Qualitative Research Practice. A Guide For Social Science Students and Researchers*, Sage, London.

Schiele, J. (2000) *Human Services and the Afrocentric Paradigm*, The Haworth Press, London.

Simon, C. & Mosavel, M. (2008) 'Key conceptual issues in the forging of community health initiatives: a South African example', *Cambridge Quarterly of Healthcare Ethics*, vol. 17, no. 2, pp. 195–205.

Social Exclusion Unit (2006) *A Sure Start to Later Life: Ending Inequalities For Older People*, Office of the Deputy Prime Minister, London.

Sue, S. (2003) 'In defense of cultural competency in psychotherapy and treatment', *American Psychologist*, vol. 58, no. 11, pp. 964–970.

US Department of Health and Human Services Office of Minority Health (2001) *National Standards For Culturally and Linguistically Appropriate Services in Health Care*, [Online] Available at: http://www.minorityhealth.hhs.gov/templates/browse.aspx?lvl = 2andlvlID = 15 (accessed 18 Jan. 2010).

Victor, C. R., Scambler, S. J., Bowling, A. N. N. & Bond, J. (2005) 'The prevalence and risk factors for loneliness in later life: a survey of older people in Great Britain', *Ageing and Society*, vol. 25, no. 3, pp. 357–375.

Warnes, A. M., Friedrich, K., Kellaher, L. & Torres, S. (2004) 'The diversity and welfare of older migrants in Europe', *Ageing and Society*, vol. 24, pp. 307–326.

Whaley, A. L. (2008) 'Cultural sensitivity and cultural competence: toward clarity of definitions in cross-cultural counselling and psychotherapy', *Counselling Psychology Quarterly*, vol. 21, pp. 215–222.

White, P. (2006) 'Migrant populations approaching old age: prospects in Europe', *Journal of Ethnic and Migration Studies*, vol. 32, pp. 1283–1300.

Wimmer, A. (2009) 'Herder's heritage and the boundary-making approach: studying ethnicity in immigrant societies', *Sociological Theory*, vol. 27, pp. 244–270.

Yan, M. C. & Wong, Y. -L. R. (2005) 'Rethinking self-awareness in cultural competence: toward a dialogic self in cross-cultural social work', *Families in Society*, vol. 86, pp. 181–188.

Yu, W. K. (2000) *Chinese Older People: A Need For Social Inclusion in Two Communities*, Policy Press, Bristol.

Yu, W. K. (2006) 'Adaptation and tradition in the pursuit of good health: Chinese people in the UK—the implications for ethnic- sensitive social work practice', *International Social Work*, vol. 49, no. 6, pp. 757–766.

Yu, W. K. (2009) 'The barriers to the effectiveness of culturally sensitive practices in health and social care services for Chinese people in Britain', *European Journal of Social Work*, vol. 12, no. 6, pp. 57–70.

Index

Note: Page numbers in *italics* represent tables
Page numbers in **bold** represent figures
Page numbers followed by 'n' refer to notes